What's So Funny About®...
Nursing?

A Creative Approach to
Celebrating Your Profession

[handwritten inscription: Rx: Laugh. Karyn Buxman]

❖ ❖ ❖

By RN, neurohumorist,
Speaker Hall of Fame inductee
Karyn Buxman

Cover design by Poole Communications
573-221-3635 | www.PooleCommunications.com

Medical studies show that people who use humor have lower levels of the stress hormones epinephrine and norepinephrine.

What's So Funny About . . .? Publishing
858-603-3133 | www.KarynBuxman.com

"A sign of a profession's maturity is its ability to laugh at itself."

~ VERA ROBINSON, PHD, RN

Disclaimer

I, Karyn Buxman, RN, MSN, CSP, CPAE, LOL, FYI, CIA, PDQ, OMG, am a neurohumorist and a nurse, but not a medical doctor—or *any* kind of doctor, for that matter. For diagnosis or treatment of any medical problem (real or imagined), consult a real doctor (*not* Doctor Seuss, Doctor Dolittle or Doctor Who). The information provided in this book is designed to provide helpful information on the subjects discussed; it is not meant to be used, nor should it be used (not even once) to diagnose or treat any medical condition. The publisher and author are not responsible for any health conditions, nor are they liable for any damages or negative consequences from any treatment or action, to any person reading or following the advice contained in this book. Readers should be aware that references are provided for informational purposes only. Readers should be aware that the medical and neurological fields evolve and change. Readers should also be aware that a spoonful of sugar makes the medicine go down.

Furthermore . . . This book is not intended to be used as a flotation device. This book is not intended for dummies. Nor for idiots. This book may be harmful if swallowed. It contains a substantial amount of non-active ingredients. Not recommended for children under 12. Batteries not included. Keep away from open flame. Colors may vary, and, in time, fade.

Storage temperature: -30C (-22F) to 40C (104F). Beware of dog. Slippery when wet. You must be present to win. Use only in well-ventilated areas. Driver does not carry cash. Tag not to be removed under penalty of law. Do not read while driving or operating heavy machinery. Do not read while sleeping. Do not fold, spindle or mutilate. Do not expose to direct sunlight. Do not puncture or incinerate. Do not pass Go. Do not collect $200.

Void where prohibited by law. Or by local custom. Or by your mom. Look both ways before crossing. No smoking. No parking. No standing.. No way. Practice safe sex. But remember that practice makes perfect. And remember to send your mother a card on her birthday. Please affix proper postage. Alcohol content is less than 12% by volume. Do not drink and drive. Do not drink and read. But it's okay to drink and watch TV. Content is rated PG-13 by the Academy for Butting Into Other People's Business. Do your civic duty and vote. Do not submerge in water. Kilroy was here. Follow your doctor's recommendations. Follow your heart. Follow the Yellow Brick Road. Good grief, Charlie Brown! Use your Zip Code! Stop! Look! And Listen! Don't over-use exclamation marks!!! Don't end sentences with prepositions. Or propositions. Don't try this at home. Seek professional advice. Where's the beef? Where's Waldo? Where oh where has my little dog gone?

Authorized personnel only. An apple a day keeps the doctor away. Do not eat of the fruit of the Tree of Knowledge of Good and Evil. Objects appear smaller than they really are. Because I said so, that's why. Fragile. This side up. Handle with care. Put your right arm in, put your right arm out, put your right arm in, and shake it all about. You do the Hokey-Pokey and you turn yourself around. (That's what it's all about.)

Watching a sitcom can increase HDL (good cholesterol) by 26%, and decrease harmful (C-reactive) proteins by 66%.

Don't run with scissors. Don't feed the animals. Don't mix plaids with stripes. Don't have a cow, man. Don't call me Shirley. Do no evil. Do unto others as you would have them do unto you. Open sesame. Open wide. Open the pod bay doors please, Hal. Houston, we have a problem. E.T. phone home. There's no place like home. Home, home on the range. How to Make Friends and Influence People. How to Succeed in Business Without Really Trying. May cause dizziness. But—thank god, will not cause constipation.

Watch for falling rocks. Watch your P's and Q's. What, me worry? Who's on first? This offer expires after 30 days. Best if used by March 31. No trespassing. Dangerous curves ahead. Deer Xing. Merry Xmas. X marks the spot. X-rated. XOXO. Riders under 54-inches must be accompanied by an adult. 25 mpg city, 43 mpg highway. 25 or 6 to 4. The answer to life, the universe, and everything: 42. Contents may settle in shipping. Results may vary. Lather. Rinse. Repeat.

This disclaimer disclaims the disclamation of its disclaimancy. And in the end . . . The love you take is equal to the love you make.

"Finally, here is a book that takes the evidence-based research of psychoneuroimmunology and makes it applicable for therapeutic benefit in patient care. As a nurse, Karyn takes the reader on a journey of the 'mind-body connection' with the use of the positive behavior—humor! And, she tells you what humor really can do for you! Karyn's approach makes the reading not only humorous but also fun and playful . . . these all translate into beneficial physiology . . . so enjoy your journey, it is different yet therapeutic because . . . 'he who laughs lasts'!"

~ LEE S. BERK, DrPH, MPH, FACSM, FAAIM, CHES, DIRECTOR, MOLECULAR RESEARCH LAB., SCHOOL OF ALLIED HEALTH; PROFESSOR, SCHOOLS OF ALLIED HEALTH, GRADUATE & MEDICINE, LOMA LINDA UNIVERSITY

"Karyn Buxman is a thought leader and master communicator in the field of applied humor. And . . . she makes me laugh!"

~ DR. HEIDI HANNA, AUTHOR OF THE SHARP SOLUTION

"What's So Funny About Nursing? is a groundbreaking book. It focuses on using healthy humor to combat stress and promote healing. Karyn Buxman is a gifted author, speaker and a nurse who shares the lighter side of the latest research in coping with illness. This is an invaluable resource for caregivers."*

~ MARY KAY MORRISON, MSED, AUTHOR OF
USING HUMOR TO MAXIMIZE LIVING

*"Five pages into this wonderful book, my cholesterol was down,
my blood pressure dropped, and I dropped 50 pounds!"*

~ ELVIS

"I wish Karyn Buxman was my mother."

~ FREUD

*"I tip my hat to 'the other humorist from Hannibal, Missouri'!
Karyn Buxman has written
The Great American Non-Fiction Advice Book!"*

~ TWAIN

*"Follow the Yellow Brick Road!
And, follow Karyn Buxman's advice!"*

~ GLINDA

*"To be (funny),
Or not to be (funny).
That is the question."*

~ HAMLET

"It's not so much about BEING funny as it is about SEEING funny."

**~ Karyn Buxman
neurohumorist**

Table of Contents

Dedications

To every nurse everywhere. Past, present and future.

And to my mom, Shirley Bradley Rapp, RN.

Acknowledgments

I would not be who I am, if it were not for nurses. I owe a huge debt to my colleagues. The work you do each and every day makes a tremendous difference. I salute you.

I've been part of the world of nursing since before I was born.* The caring, compassion, and grace-under-fire I learned from my family and my colleagues has served me well in all walks of my life.

Here's a high-five to my colleagues, mentors and friends at the Association for Applied & Therapeutic Humor. We are making the world a better place one

---

* My mother, a nurse anesthetist, used to laugh and say that I accompanied her to work until the day before she went into labor! This book wouldn't exist if it weren't for my mom, Shirley Bradley Rapp, RN, pilot, mentor. Oh! And I'd better thank my dad, too! I guess I wouldn't even *exist* if he and my mom hadn't, um, gotten together. So here's to Dr. LaMoine Rapp, the beloved family practitioner in Mark Twain's hometown, Hannibal, Missouri. Oh! And thanks to my amazing little sister, Dr. Susan Rapp, too!

laugh at a time. And a special shout-out to Mary Kay Morrison and the Humor Academy for giving me the shove I needed to get the "What's So Funny About... ?" project into high gear.

Kudos to Dr. Lee Berk, Dr. Michael Miller, Dr. William Fry, Dr. Paul McGhee, and the numerous others who have conducted the clinical research behind this book. You are making a tremendous difference in the lives of people around the planet.

Thanks to my grad school (Go Mizzou!) advisors, Virginia Bzdek, Mandy Manderino, and Sherry Mustapha. You believed in me and encouraged me to take that first step so many years ago, in spite of the fact that most everyone else saw research into therapeutic humor as "not professional enough." Your support has been like a pebble cast into the water. I really want you to know that your influence is now global in scope.

To Peter and all the regulars at the Pacific Bean Coffee Shop: Thanks for keeping me well-caffeinated during this book project. I haven't drunk that much coffee since I worked in surgery!

To Dr. Vera Robinson, who, because of her pioneering work in therapeutic humor back in the 1970s, was lovingly referred to as the "Fairy Godmother of Humor"; and to my beloved colleagues from the hilarious (and infamous) *Journal of Nursing Jocularity* back in the

1990s: Doug Fletcher, Patty Wooten, Fran London, John Wise, Bob Quick—we tread where others dared not go. We took our licks and kept on laughing.

To Sally and her terrific crew at Poole Communications. Thanks for making this book—and me-—look good!

A huge thank you to my editor Cindy Potts, whose talent, tenacity, and twisted sense of humor have made this entire "What's So Funny About... ?" project a blast!

And of course, this book would not be here were it not for my incredibly-patient-mildly-brilliant-and-oh-so-romantic-husband, Greg Godek. *[Who has more fun than you and me?]* *[Nobody!]*

Foreword

by Patty Wooten, RN, BSN, CIC

What's so funny about nursing? One answer is: "Nothing!" And an equally valid answer is "A whole lot!" It all depends on your perspective. And that's what this book is all about: Perspective.

My friend and fellow nurse Karyn Buxman is a member of a special sorority of nurses who understands the seriousness of our profession, *and* the silliness, outrageousness and craziness of our lives as professional caregivers. Perspective leads to insight and wisdom. And Karyn's talent is using humor to help us gain perspective.

Nursing is serious and challenging work. A nurse needs to be smart, strong, organized, fearless, persuasive, tolerant, creative, intuitive, flexible, perceptive . . . and the list goes on and on. Believe me, I know this to be true. For the last 40 years I've been a nurse in intensive care, med-surg, public health, long term care, hospice, PACU, telemetry, and infection prevention. Many days I felt frustrated, insulted, threatened, abused, overwhelmed and exhausted—and those were the *good* days. Yet, never was there a day when I doubted that I had made a difference in someone's life. How many professions offer that opportunity?

I'm sure every nurse has heard, "Oh, you're a nurse! Wow, I could never do that. How do you cope?" We all cope in different ways on different days. We cry, we pray and sometimes we scream (usually in the car on the way home). Most nurses have experienced the stress relieving effects of laughter. Many of us have said to a colleague, after a robust shared laugh, "Thanks, I really needed that!" After a good laugh we feel lighter, stronger and ready to face the next challenge. I believe that's why God made our job so funny.

What's So Funny About . . . Nursing? is a vital resource for every nurse. This book is a practical guide to finding and creating more opportunities for laughter right alongside the challenges we face each day. You will learn what humor and laughter can do for your physical health, emotional balance, social interaction and communication skills.

Karyn Buxman is one of the funniest people I know. And she is uniquely qualified to clarify the therapeutic value of humor and laughter. As a nurse, she understands the reality of nursing. For the last 25 years she has researched humor, collaborated with experts around the world, and helped more than a quarter million people appreciate the value of humor and laughter. This book will help you discover and appreciate what's so funny about nursing.

PATTY WOOTEN, RN, BSC, CIC

NURSE HUMORIST
AUTHOR OF *COMPASSIONATE LAUGHTER*

Introduction

It's no secret that I think nurses are amazing—it's really blindingly obvious, actually. After the presentation of my nursing masters thesis made my advisors laugh,* and I discovered that I was funny [who knew?!], I dedicted myself to sharing the benefits of "applied humor" to nurses worldwide. Since then I've spoken to more than 100,000 nurses in most American states and several foreign countries.

Nurses have a calling, not merely a career. Being a professional caregiver is fulfilling, exhilirating, challenging and exhausting! You've got to be able to think on your feet, recognize and respond to potential complications, and advocate for the patient—all while providing the best possible care and maintaining a positive relationship with your healthcare colleagues.

Nursing is an amazing profession, and nurses are amazing people. But let's not kid ourselves. This is hard work we're doing. There are tremendous demands on our physical, mental, and emotional resources. We need support.

---

*My masters thesis was *about* humor and healthcare, but it was not intended to *be* humorous.

Support isn't always forthcoming. The healthcare system is under increasing pressure to do more-and-more with less-and-less. Budgets are tight. Good leadership teams—teams that want to provide their nurses with every available resource to enhance morale and boost performance—often don't have the money to make it happen.

"It would not be possible to praise nurses too highly."
~ STEPHEN AMBROSE

That's why humor is so important. Laughter is an amazing therapeutic tool for you, your patients, and the healthcare team you work with. There are physical, emotional, and organizational benefits associated with the use of humor—and best of all, it's free! The purposeful and deliberate cultivation of humor is one way to ensure better patient outcomes, enhance individual professional performance, and boost team morale.

You don't need to spend any money to access humor. You don't need to buy anything to laugh. [It helps, of course, to buy this book. Ha! Multiple copies help even *more*, because then you can share the laughs with a friend!] In an environment of increasing demands and dwindling resources, humor is the answer.

You may be thinking to yourself, "But I'm not *funny*. Can you *teach* me to be funny?" Well, yes. I could teach you a short comedy bit that might serve you every now and then. But it's not about *being* funny as much as it is about *seeing* funny. If you can "*see* funny," then the "*be* funny" will fall into place.

Odds are that you already have a sense of humor. The fact that you've picked up and are reading this book means that the chances are even better that it's a *good* sense of humor. But it's possible to improve and focus your humor skills to make them stronger and more effective. That way, when you really need a good laugh, you'll be able to have one—guaranteed!

So fasten your seatbelt, put your tray in the upright and locked position, and let's go!

YOURS IN LAUGHTER!
KARYN BUXMAN, RN, MSN, CSP, CPAE,
NEUROHUMORIST

RN: REGISTERED NURSE

MSN: MASTER OF SCIENCE IN NURSING

CSP: CERTIFIED SPEAKING PROFESSIONAL

CPAE: THE SPEAKER HALL OF FAME (THE OSCARS OF THE SPEAKING PROFESSION)

NEUROHUMORIST: ONE WHO COMBINES APPLIED HUMOR WITH CUTTING-EDGE NEUROSCIENCE

THIS BOOK IS INTENDED FOR NURSES ONLY.
ALTHOUGH 99.9% OF THE HUMOR CONTAINED
HEREIN IS BOTH UNDERSTANDABLE AND APPROPRIATE
FOR THE REASONABLY-INTELLLIGENT AND
LIBERAL-MINDED LAYPERSON—
IT'S THE REMAINING 0.1% OF THE CONTENT THAT
MAY CAUSE NON-PROFESSIONALS TO EXPERIENCE
HEART PALPITATIONS, DIZZINESS AND/OR
MORAL OUTRAGE.
THUS, THE READER MAY WANT TO CARRY THIS BOOK
IN A BROWN PAPER WRAPPER.

"Humor is power."

~ KARYN BUXMAN, NEUROHUMORIST

Chapter 1
What's NOT So Funny About Nursing?

12 hour shifts . . . Doctors with attitude . . . Cranky co-workers . . . Frequent flyers . . . Non-compliant patients . . . Frustrated administrators . . . Antibiotic-resistant superbugs . . . Healthcare reform . . . Disorganized supply closets . . . Dwindling budgets . . . Increasing workloads . . . Bad hospital coffee.

Not funny. Not funny. Not funny.

How many of your friends went through years and years of higher education so they can go into work in the morning and be puked on? How many of them work in an environment in which a mistake can actually *kill someone*?

No matter what type of nursing you practice, there's one thing that's absolutely true: Nursing is hard. Let's talk about that for a moment. It's a conversation that doesn't happen as often as it needs to.

Nursing has its own distinct culture—which has its positives and its negatives. You can't beat the nursing culture for the closeness of team members. Working long hours in a demanding environment creates some of the strongest bonds in healthcare. I can't begin to tell you how many nurses tell me that it is the support of their colleagues that keeps them hanging in there, day after day.

> **Humor provides measurable physiological benefits.**
>
> **Laughter relieves social tension.**
>
> **Laughter relieves internal tension, too!**

On the other hand, there's this weird bravado that permeates nursing culture. We give challenges the silent treatment—we just don't discuss the things that really bother us. One of the things we don't talk about is what nursing does to nurses.

Being a front line healthcare provider is tough work. No matter what setting you work in—a hospital, a physician's office, a school, a correctional facility, a military hospital—you are the ultimate patient advocate. In your hands is the safety and well-being of your patients—and sometimes they're actively working against your efforts to keep them safe and healthy! Keeping things safe and moving requires the highest order of multi-tasking; your intense focus is required on multiple fronts. The sheer breadth of knowledge it takes to do your job is staggering. All of this takes a physical and emotional toll.

What is this doing to *you?*

As a nurse, you're under a lot of stress. Nursing may not be *the* most stressful profession in the world—that "honor" may belong to air traffic controllers. Or maybe single moms. But nursing is pretty near the top of the list. You may not feel this stress all of the time—one of the great things about human nature is that we can acclimate ourselves to even the most outrageous of situations—but the stress has a real and dramatic impact on your physical and emotional health.

Here are some of the highlights (or rather, low-lights):

- Heart health: Cardiovascular disease and hypertension are both linked to high stress levels. Heart disease is currently the number one cause of death— for both men and women—in America, affecting nearly 50% of the population.

- Respiratory health: People who have high levels of stress experience COPD and asthma more often than people who report lower stress levels.

- Digestive tract: Stress can work havoc on the GI system. Whether it's ulcers, gastritis, ulcerative colitis or IBS, stress can really make your stomach hurt. GI conditions are one of the most common stress-related complaints. Over the past two decades, we've seen procedures on the GI tract become steadily more and more common—surely a sign of our stressful times.

- Body aches and pains: High stress levels contribute to pain throughout the body, especially in the shoulders, neck, and lower back. For some people, lots of stress means they experience painful twinges, twitches, or ticks. Nurses have a high incidence of temporal mandibular joint disease—or TMJ—from grinding and/or clenching their teeth. [Who? Me?!]

- Reproductive issues: Stress can really interfere with your love life—and any plans you may have for a future family. Research has tied high stress levels to impotence and infertility, as well as menstrual disorders and recurrent vaginal infections.

- Hair loss: Stress can make you go bald! —Or lose handfuls of your hair. [So much for a good hair day!]

- Mental health: Stress isn't good for our mental health, either. Anxiety, depression, irritability and insomnia are often reported by people experiencing high levels of stress. High stress levels can also manifest in aggressive, anti-social behavior. That's why it is important to find effective ways to continually manage stress.

- Aging: And just to top things off, some research suggests that stress even make us get older faster! [We're not talking laugh lines here!]

"Wrinkles should merely indicate where smiles have been."

~ MARK TWAIN

I have to admit that being stressed-out isn't particularly fun or humorous. There's no point in making light of the serious side of our challenging profession. But while the stress that comes with nursing really isn't funny, the *experiences* you have while being a nurse can be absolutely hysterical.

The premise of this book—borne out by scientific research—is that humor has many practical benefits that nurses can use to benefit themselves, their patients and the team of professionals they're such a vital part of. Techniques of applied humor have made a positive difference in healthcare settings across the country and around the world.

It's life-changing. It's proven. It's easy. It's fun.

So what are we waiting for??

"Humor restores the human touch, the caring, to the highly technical, potentially dehumanizing world of healthcare."

~ VERA ROBINSON, PhD, RN

"If we took what we now know about laughter and bottled it, it would require FDA approval."

~ DR. LEE BERK, RESEARCHER, PSYCHONEUROIMMUNOLOGIST

Chapter 2
What Humor Can Do for You

Now it's time for some GOOD news! While we've known since Biblical times that laughter makes us feel better—"A merry heart doeth good like a medicine." (Proverbs 17:22)—science is finally starting to *prove* it! The positive effects of laughter are evident in almost every body system.

In Medieval times it was thought that if the body's fluids (known then as "umors") were in balance, one was of good temperament—or healthy. That's where the phrase "having a good sense of humor" came from. The umors were yellow bile, black bile, blood, and lymph.

Throughout the Middle Ages, the practice of medicine was more art than science. And as art goes—well, let's just say you should be glad you didn't live back in the days of yore! The following is from a *Saturday Night Live* skit, with comedian Steve Martin playing Theodoric of York, a doctor/barber:

> *"You know, medicine is not an exact science,*
> *but we are learning all the time.*
> *Why, just fifty years ago, they thought a disease*
> *like your daughter's*
> *was caused by demonic possession or witchcraft.*
> *But nowadays we know that Isabelle is suffering from an*
> *imbalance of bodily humors,*
> *perhaps caused by a toad or a small dwarf*
> *living in her stomach."*

We now know that umor, or humor, isn't a body fluid at all. [And it's pretty rare indeed to find a toad or small dwarf living in anyone's stomach.] But I digress . . .

So, if humor isn't a body fluid—exactly what *is* it? Here's the most *concise* definition . . .

"Humor is whatever people find funny."

~ Elaine Pasquali

Hmmm . . . This may the most *concise* definition—but is it the most *insightful* definition?

How about a *psychoanalyst's* view? Sigmund Freud's definition is . . .

> *"Humor is a coping mechanism*
> *that allows persons to reduce tension and anxiety*
> *by expressing obscene or hostile impulses*
> *in a socially acceptable manner."*

That's rather intense, isn't it?! It certainly contains some truth. But is it really helpful?? Perhaps not.

How about a *comedian's* opinion? Groucho Marx said . . .

> *"Humor is reason gone mad."*

Hmmm . . . Short is good. Funny is good. But perhaps this is a little *too* pithy.

How about an *educator's* thoughts? Joel Goodman, founder of The HUMORProject, weighs in with . . .

> *"Humor is a childlike perspective*
> *in an otherwise serious adult reality."*

Hmmm . . . I *like* this one!

And how about a *psychologist's* point-of-view? One therapist, Steve Sultanoff, Ph.D. says . . .

"Humor is the INTELLECTUAL mindset expressed
through the EMOTIONAL feelings of mirth
and the PHYSICAL expression of laughter."

Hmmm . . . I like this one, *too*! It links the intellectual, emotional and physical modalities with the three elements that comprise humor: Mindset, mirth and laughter.

And finally, perhaps we should consider a defintion from a *neurohumorist:*

"Humor is a feeling of delight, wonder or release—
that comes from surprise, perspective or insight."

Oh, wait! That's *my* definition of humor. [I'm rather partial to it, but I won't insist! I've given you six definitions, so you you can choose the one that works best for you, or mix-and-match them to create your *own* definition of humor.]

Delight. Wonder. Release. I love the idea of looking at life through the eyes of a child; they have such a sense of fun and playfulness [which we seem to lose as we get older, more serious, and more "professional"]. And perspective is the underpinning of all reframing—our ability to *see* funny, and ultimately our ability to just be happier.

True story . . . from the Karyn Buxman Archives:

It was eight o'clock on a Monday morning. In my haste to get myself ready for the work day, I'd temporarily forgotten about my seven-year-old son. A rhythmic thumping noise coming from upstairs brought him back to mind.

A mom-on-a-mission, I ran up the stairs. As I approached Adam's room I could feel the *Whomp! Whomp! Whomp!* vibrating through the walls.

"What in the world—?!" I wondered.

I opened his door and saw Adam—wearing nothing but his underwear and a big smile—jumping up and down on his bed . . . singing and dancing . . . swinging his shirt over and around his head . . . with enthusiastic kicks accenting the beat.

"What do you think you're doing, young man?" I demanded.

Adam stopped mid-jump, grinned a huge grin, and with the wisdom of Yoda, said, "Don't-ya-think-getting-dressed-in-the-morning-oughta-be-more-*fun*, Mom?!"

Let's think about this . . . What if *getting dressed* in the morning *could* be more fun? What if *getting up in the morning* could be more fun? What if *going to work* could be more fun?! By playing with our perspective, we can create a happier experience—for ourselves, for our families, and for our patients.

—————

Four of the main sources of humor are surprise, derailment, delight and [believe-it-or-not] pain and discomfort.

1. Surprise

Humor can come from surprise. "Boo!" "Gotcha!" "April Fool!" When situations aren't what we expect them to be, or people act in an altogether unforeseeable fashion, our first response is often to laugh.

2. Derailment

Humor can come from "derailment"—the sudden twist, the confounding of expectation. The new resident turns to greet you—and she's wearing a red clown nose.

3. Delight

Humor can come from pure delight. Opening Christmas presents. Dinner with good friends. A child with a helium balloon. [Children experience much more delight than adults do. Perhaps we should take note.]

4. Pain

Humor can come from pain and discomfort. ("Huh?!!") *The Three Stooges. Candid Camera. America's Funniest Home Videos*. People don't laugh about having too much money, a perfect marriage, or a good hair day—they laugh about their nagging mother-in-law, their obstinant teenager, their aggravating co-workers. Nurses also laugh about body fluids, death and dismemberment [but more on *that* later!].

––––––––––

There has been a lot of serious research into what makes us laugh—and what laughter does for us. These studies come from a field of research called psychoneuroimmunology. Yes, it's a mouthful, but as the study of humor gets serious [Ha!], we have been moving from *qualitative* research (lots and lots—and lots, of anecdotal evidence), toward *quantitative* research (including controlled studies and electrodes and brain scans). "Psycho-neuro-immunology . . . where psycho = mind; neuro = nervous system; and immunology = immune system)—which is sometimes referred to as the mind-body connection. Some experts throw in the endocrine system, too, making this the study of "psychoneuroimmunoendocrinology." [How many points is that in *Words with Friends*?]

For simplicity [and sanity], I'll refer to this as PNI from here on out. Here are the highlights of that research . . .

What Humor Can Do for Your *Body*

Humor and laughter have many positive effects on your body. PNI has illuminated many of the strong connections between the experience of laughter and improved wellness. Research has been conducted on the humor-health connection as it pertains to almost every body system: The cardiovascular, respiratory, immune, musculo-skeletal, endocrine, reproductive, nervous and digestive systems have all been studied, and the work done there has been revelatory.

Let's Get to the Heart of the Matter

Humor can help you bring your cholesterol levels down—and it's way more fun than eating bowls of oatmeal and granola! In a study conducted by psychoneuroimmunologist Dr. Lee Berk, and his endocrinologist and diabetes specialist colleague, Dr. Stanley Tan, participants spent half an hour a day watching movies or sitcoms that they found humorous. As a result, the participants' levels of LDL decreased, while HDL increased, and harmful C-reactive proteins declined.

When was the last time you heard that watching TV could actually *make you healthier*?! Another way you can really give your heart a boost is by playing the ICU Game: Any time you see an error on a medical TV show (*Nurse Jackie* and *Grey's Anatomy* are GREAT for this!) that would result in the patient spending the rest of his short, short life in the ICU, get up and do 25 jumping jacks. You could have the heart of an Olympian in less than one season!

While you *do* want to reduce your harmful cholesterol, and lower your risk for cardiovascular disease, you probably *don't* want to do two-dozen jumping jacks between every set of commercials!

Laughing is a lot less work. Reducing cholesterol is one example of how humor can do more than just make you *feel* better: Humor can help you *be* better.

"The old saying that 'laughter is the best medicine,' definitely appears to be true when it comes to protecting your heart," says Michael Miller, M.D., Director of the Center for Preventive Cardiology at the University of Maryland Medical Center and a professor of medicine at the University of Maryland School of Medicine. "The ability to laugh—either naturally or as a learned behavior—may have important implications in societies such as the U.S. where heart disease remains the number one killer . . . We know that exercising, eating foods low in saturated fat, and not smoking will reduce the risk of heart disease. Perhaps regular, hearty laughter should be added to the list."

Improve Your Vascular Health

Laughter helps lower your blood pressure and increase circulation. Maintaining optimal circulation is absolutely critical. It's important for you to keep the blood flowing to your extremities. Circulation is important because a constant, fresh supply of oxygenated blood keeps your energy level up—and if there's one thing every nurse needs, it's lots of energy!

A recent study by Dr. Miller advances our understanding of the mind-body connection. His research shows for the first time that laughter is linked to the healthy functioning of blood vessels. Laughter appears to cause the tissue that forms the inner lining of blood vessels, the endothelium, to dilate in order to increase blood flow.

"We know it works." Dr. Miller told me. There's an apparent relationship between mental stress and vasoconstriction. And no one appreciates healthy circulation like a nurse does! We don't want our blood vessels tight and constricted. Nothing makes us happier than for them to be wide open, flexible healthy highways for the transport of oxygenated blood. "The endothelium is one of the most basic cardiac mechanisms. The fact that it is highly responsive to robust laughter means we have a real story here. And there's no downside to laughter!" adds Dr. Miller.

Blood Glucose Control

"Why should I worry about blood sugar? I don't have diabetes!" But did you know that 1 in 10 Americans has diabetes? The right lifestyle choices can help minimize that risk. And let's face it: When your lunch consists of a Diet Coke and a Snickers Bar, you're not making the world's best lifestyle choices.

So bring on the humor! Humor can help lower the increase in blood sugar you experience after eating a meal. A recent study shows that people who watched a brief comedy show after eating, had lower glucose values than those who did not see the program. Pretty sweet!

Other studies show that laughing lowers your levels of the stress hormones cortisol and adrenaline. Cortisol increases insulin resistance, while adrenaline tells your liver to pump more glucose into your blood. The combined effect can be a lasting reduction in blood glucose levels.

"While there is no reason to expect humor to be helpful in PREVENTING diabetes, it IS helpful in MANAGING it."

~ DR. PAUL MCGHEE,
HUMOR, THE LIGHTER PATH TO RESILIENCE & HEALTH

Immune System

Nurses have raised infection control to an art form. We'll preserve the integrity of a sterile field by any means necessary—and that's not Hollywood hyperbole. Protecting the patient is a top priority, but maintaining our own health in the face of some frightening emerging pathogens is a very, very close second. [No one wants to wind up written into the medical literature!]

Still, in the back of your mind, the worry remains: "Is my *own* immune system strong enough to deal with everything I face in the healthcare setting?"

Laughter is a low-tech way to augment your natural immune response. Humor and laughter have been found to significantly increase spontaneous lymphocyte blastogenesis, a natural killer cell activity, as well as stimulate Immunoglobulin A, which is especially helpful in combatting respiratory infections. Pretty significant benefits from a few chuckles, eh?!

Gastrointestinal System

Remember back in nursing school when we learned that walking and moving patients around would improve peristalsis? Well, laughing can do the same thing. Our abdominal muscles massage our internal organs when we have a good belly laugh, which stimulates peristalsis and enhances digestion. This can be good for patients who may not have the ability to ambulate. It's also good news for nurses who, after a twelve hour shift, don't feel one bit like ambulating!

"A person who belly-laughs doesn't bellyache."
~ SUSAN THURMAN, ENGLISH TEACHER

In a perfect world, all nurses would eat healthy meals, at regular intervals, at times roughly in alignment with the rest of humanity. It turns out that we don't necessarily live in a perfect world. I don't mean to shock you, but some nurses don't always eat the healthiest meals. In other words, no, you can't find all four food groups in the vending machine. [And no, grape-flavored bubble gum does *not* count as a fruit!] Meals are eaten on the go, at strange hours—or are sometimes skipped entirely. This can create havoc on your GI system.

Humor can help. Not as much as a well-timed tuna sandwich, perhaps. But I've found that the ability to access laughter quickly can be a tremendous asset when admissions keep rolling in, and the chances of your sitting down for a meal are smaller than your chances of winning the lottery!

Pain Management

Researchers have found that humor helps with pain management. It does so by increasing pain tolerance levels and by distraction. Chronic neck, back and joint pain are part of too many nurses' lives. Knee, ankle and hip complaints are common as well. Whether the pain is sporadic or chronic, experiencing it adds an unwanted toll to your already full day. Effective pain management really should be part of your daily routine.

Laughter lowers blood pressure, decreases muscle tension, and reduces anxiety and inflammation. This helps relieve pain throughout the body. And less pain results in better sleep. [And what nurse couldn't benefit from a better night's—or day's—sleep?!]

The Ohio State University Medical Center provides patients with a handout detailing the value of humor in pain management. By providing a distraction, humor shifts one's focus away from the pain and onto whatever you're laughing at. It doesn't *eliminate* the pain, but it helps you deal with it more effectively. Humor reduces the prominent position pain plays in your day.

What Humor Can Do for Your *Emotions*

Being a nurse requires you to have exceptional emotional elasticity. You're deeply invested in your patients, focused on achieving the best possible outcomes—every time. Sometimes this happens. Sometimes it doesn't. There are good days, and there are bad days.

You have to go back to work after the bad days. That takes strength and fortitude. It takes what scientists call emotional resiliency—the ability to "bounce back" to a centered, stable emotional state relatively quickly after a shock or disruption of expected events. Some nurses are better at this than others.

Researchers who have been working on understanding why some people are more emotionally resilient than others have discovered that emotional resiliency may not be an innate quality. You're not necessarily born with the ability to roll with life's punches. Instead, emotional resiliency develops as a result of identifiable processes we can choose to engage in.

And so, just for you, I researched resilience . . . and found the American Psychological Association's . . .

Top 10 Ways to Build Resilience

10. Maintain good relationships with close family members, friends and others.

9. Avoid seeing crises or stressful events as unbearable problems.

8. Accept circumstances that cannot be changed.

7. Develop realistic goals and move toward them.

6. Take decisive actions in adverse situations.

5. Look for opportunities of self-discovery after a struggle with loss.

4. Develop self-confidence.

3. Keep a long-term perspective and consider the stressful event in a broader context.

2. Maintain a hopeful outlook, expect good things, and visualize your wishes.

1. Take care of your mind and body; exercise regularly; pay attention to your own needs and feelings.

Laughter definitely fits into this equation. As a way to take care of one's mind and body, humor makes it easier to maintain your emotional stability and well-being while enabling you to provide the best possible patient care. Humor makes you feel good. It lifts your mood and results in a more positive overall outlook. This positive outlook is a great resource to have when you've just been chewed-up and spit-out by an uptight doctor or an upset family member. But that's not all that humor can do.

Humor also delivers the following valuable emotional benefits . . .

Provides an Outlet for Anger

Life is not fair—just ask any nurse! Bad things happen, and this makes us angry—angry at the causes of the bad things, angry that bad things happen at all, angry at the world where the bad things have become all too common. There are times when anger is an appropriate and even healthy response.

But it's hard to be a good nurse while you're angry. The healthcare environment demands a clarity of thought inconsistent with intense anger. If you're so angry you can't see straight, that's not a good thing—for you, for your colleagues, or for your patients.

Getting angry is natural. But *staying* angry is a choice. The emotional experience of anger provokes biochemical changes within the body. These changes manifest in many ways. A churning stomach, a blinding headache, pounding blood pressure and/or chronic fatigue. Raise your hand if you've experienced any of these. During the past week.

Anger accumulates. Anger builds. Anger is the

kudzu vine in your emotional garden: Once it puts down roots and starts growing, there's just no stopping it—unless you take action. Humor stops anger. If you want to control your rage and cut down the kudzu of hostility that's keeping you up at night, try laughing.

"It is impossible for you to be angry and laugh at the same time. Anger and laughter are mutually exclusive—and you have the power to choose either."

~ WAYNE DYER

It turns out that laughter is a very effective mechanism for processing negative emotions. Even the most bitter laughter is a form of gaining a new perspective on a situation. Many comedians assert that their best material comes out of the times in their lives when they were angriest. And while people will run like the building is on fire when a complainer approaches, humor can be a socially acceptable—and enjoyable—way for people to vent.

Humor provides a way for us to *express* our anger, rather than *repressing* it. Try as you might, it is impossible to ignore feelings of anger in the long run. Add to that the fact that other people around you—whom you spend hours with every day—are having their *own* experiences with anger, and the whole thing can be a recipe for disaster. It's important to acknowledge that we have, at times, feelings of frustration and rage.

But we can't always *act* on our feelings of frustration and rage. There are laws against that type of thing! And doing *nothing* about it isn't really a good option, either. Repressed anger and frustration can make your stress levels sky-rocket. In addition to that, chronic, sustained anger has been identified

> *Neurobiologists have proven that humor provides benefits to the cardiovascular, respiratory, immune, and musculo-skeletal systems.*

as a contributing factor in heart disease, high blood pressure and stroke.

What to *do* with anger? You can avoid it. You can deny it. Or you can redirect it—by using humor. This redirection can defuse a lot of rage, bringing with it a sense of calm, relief and a fresh perspective. The underlying circumstances that made us angry still exist, but after we've laughed we're better prepared to address those circumstances.

It feels good to laugh at problems, if only for a moment. This doesn't mean closing our eyes to reality. Instead, laughter allows us to reframe the issue and look at it anew. Sometimes a change in perspective presents the information we need to move past the anger.

*"Laughter gives us distance.
It allows us to step back from an event,
deal with it, and then move on."*

~ BOB NEWHART

Reduces Stress

Humor is a powerful tool for stress reduction. As we talked about earlier, stress is one of the biggest challenges associated with nursing. Stress has all kinds of negative physical and emotional ramifications that are better off avoided. For that reason, we need to minimize our stress levels.

Signs of Stress (The Nurse's Version)

• Everyone around you has an attitude problem.

• Every time you see an empty patient's bed you have an overwhelming desire to lie down on it.

• When you see an episode of *Dexter*, your reaction is, "That's my life . . . except with less blood."

• You feel like the author of the book *I've Got One Nerve Left and You're Standing On It.*

- You eat a one-pound bag of M&Ms at one sitting.

- You add chocolate chips to your Caesar salad.

- You swipe candy from patients' bedside tables while they're sleeping.

- You put straws in specimen containers.

Is humor the *best* coping mechanism? I guess that's a matter of opinion! But humor is certainly one of the *healthiest*. You can get over a bad day at work with a bottle of red wine—or two!—but that takes a toll on your system. Comfort eating, retail therapy, and behavior-based addictions like gambling, may feel good temporarily. In the long run, however, you might not be so thrilled with how things turn out. Laughter lets you have lots of fun—and you'll still be thin, sober and solvent in the morning.

By relieving anxiety and tension, humor provides a healthy escape from reality, and lightens the heaviness related to the aspects of caregiving that really weigh you down.

What Humor Can Do for You *Socially*

One of my favorite things about being a nurse, a humorist, and a professional speaker is the time I get to spend with fellow nurses. It is my honor and privilege to hear about the triumphs, the challenges, and the funny moments you face.

But it's heartbreaking to hear about the difficulties we nurses have getting along with each other. Lateral hostility is a real problem in the nursing world. Kathleen Bartholomew, RN, MN, has conducted groundbreaking work, examining how interpersonal relationships affect the healthcare workplace. Nurses are being bullied by physicians, by patients, and by each other.

This needs to stop. Making it stop will require massive, systematic changes to our culture and to the healthcare system. I think we're in the very early stages of seeing those changes happen—but you still have to go to work in the meantime.

Humor can play many roles in our response to bullying behavior. In a perfect world, we'd all be empowered to challenge bullying behavior whenever we see it. Pragmatically, there are times when confronting a bully directly can have personal, professional, or economic consequences that are beyond what you're willing to pay. During these times, humor can serve as a comfort and solace, helping preserve emotional resiliency.

Viktor Frankl, author of *Man's Search for Meaning*, survived Nazi concentration camps during World War II. He later wrote of the experience, "To discover that there was any semblance of art in a concentration camp must be surprise enough for an outsider, but he may be even more astonished to hear that one could find a sense of humor there as well; of course, only the faint trace of one, and then only for a few seconds or minutes. Humor was another of the soul's weapons in the fight for self-preservation. It is well known that humor, more than anything else in the human make-up, can afford an aloofness and an ability to rise above any situation, even if only for a few seconds."

Humor can be useful during those times when you need to address problem behaviors. Humor is power.

> The new nurse had been forewarned about the neurologist who liked to pick on new staff. So when he charged onto the unit and fired a bunch of questions at her, she had all the answers.
>
> The fact that she was prepared seemed to make the doc all the more cantankerous. Finally he barked at her, "How *long* have you been a nurse?"

She looked at him and asked, "What time is it?"

He glared at her. She smiled and raised her eyebrows. They both burst into laughter.

And he never tried to bully her again.

Fighting Isolation

Nursing has always been an isolating profession, and I think the situation is getting worse. That's not good news. When we feel lonely, we are more prone to depression and anxiety—not a good combination.

There are several reasons for this sense of isolation. One is the simply the nature of the job. We're busy every single minute of our shift. You've got more to do than time in which to do it. There's simply no time to do anything but focus on the job at hand. Everyone you work with is busy too, which makes a tough situation even tougher. And the trend from 8-hour to 12-hour shifts means that there's less time to socialize after work.

The other reason nurses are feeling more isolated has nothing to do with your job, and everything to do with your smartphone. Social media has been around for nearly two decades now, which means that many younger nurses have spent more time *texting* than they have *talking*! And we older—I mean, more mature—

nurses are not immune to the magnetic pull of our smartphones, either.

It has been documented that there has been a significant and widespread deterioration in Americans' collective communication skills over the past decade and-a-half. Is there anything more frustrating than a patient who wants you to wait for her to finish her call before you begin your exam? I'm still not sure what to think of individuals who Tweet mid-procedure. The plethora of small screens in our lives has significantly affected our ability to communicate face-to-face.

Is this impact negative or positive? The jury is still out. A study conducted by The University of Gothenburg in Sweden focused on finding the link between self-esteem and Facebook usage. Researchers found that as Facebook interaction increased, self-esteem decreased. On the other hand, a 2009 study published in the journal *Cyberpsychology, Behavior and Social Networking* reports a significant *rise* in self-esteem among Facebook users.

Being mindful of our social media usage and finding ways to connect more regularly—and laugh with!—others in person will have a positive effect on your personal and professional life.

"Laughter is the shortest distance between two people."
~ Victor Borge

Humor has been found to strengthen existing relationships [which is good if you *like* the people you know!]. Regular use of humor is thought to make us more attractive to other people, which can increase your social circle and your base of support [and this is good news if you *don't* like the people you currently know!].

In the next section, we'll take a look at how that works.

Levels the Playing Field

As nurses, we occupy a unique place in the healthcare community. We're not doctors—the folks who generally get most of the credit. Our role is both vital, and largely behind-the-scenes. This can make it difficult at times to form positive relationships with the other people we work with. Humor can help smooth over those differences.

A little humor helps to break down awkward moments between people. It doesn't matter what race you are, what gender or what religion you are, or how much money you make . . . If something is funny, people laugh.

Laughter reduces social hierarchies, making it easier for people from different social circles, and different life circumstances, to connect with each other. Whether it's doctor/nurse, administrator/staff, or nurse/patient, when we can laugh together, communication becomes easier. And that's important.

What Humor Can Do for Your *Communications*

Gets Your Message Across

One of the first times it became evident to me that humor can help get your point across, I was teaching student nurses about orthostatic hypotension.

In great detail I described the effects of decreased blood pressure resulting from getting up too quickly and the physiological effects of anoxia on the brain. In a closed classroom with no windows, following the lunch period, I gazed around the classroom at 28 blank faces. In desperation I jumped up, pointed to my head and shouted, "May Day! May Day! All systems down! We don't have enough oxygen up here so we're going down!" and then plopped to the floor.

Startled, the students bolted upright and burst into laughter. During the next test, ripples of laughter could be heard as students reached the question on orthostatic hypotension. I could hear the words "May Day! May Day!" being whispered. Not one student missed that question.

Humor is a helpful communications tool because it grabs people's attention. Teachers, preachers, speakers, and politicians all agree, if you want to get people listening, get them laughing. People enjoy laughing. And when you inject humor into your communications, people pay more attention and they loosen-up—and this helps them hear your serious messages better.

Humor can also serve as a safety net, for when you get into awkward or difficult conversations. The ability to frame topics as potentially humorous material allows you to bring up serious subjects while "testing the waters" with people. If they respond well to your humorous tone, it becomes easier to move the conversation forward and address larger issues. Even humor that *doesn't* work can spark meaningful, much-needed conversations. Even a joke that falls flat can be a door-opener. You might shrug your shoulders, chuckle and say, "You know, I never *could* tell a joke. But you know, the issue of _____ is no joke!"

Humor can enhance important communication, whether it's with a patient, a colleague or a friend.

Defuses Difficult Situations

The healthcare environment is the setting for many difficult, tense moments. There are many ways to deal with difficult situations—but one that's frequently overlooked is humor.

When things get tense, whether it's dealing with a red-faced doctor in a full-fledged-meltdown, or a garden-variety personality conflict, humor can diffuse the anger, relieve the tension, and level the playing field. Good communicators—like successful comedians or politicians (or comedians who *become* politicians; see: Al Franken)—will have a list of laugh lines, or "saver lines," that they can pull out when things unexpectedly go awry.

"Language was created so we could communicate. Humor was created so we could complain."

~ KARYN BUXMAN, NEUROHUMORIST

You never know when you're going need them, but if you can come up with your own saver lines, you can give yourself more power and control by being proactive. Try this: Collect humorous lines and quotes you can use to stop angry bluster in its tracks. If people start laughing, they stop yelling—and that's good news for everyone. Here are some saver lines you can use to get started:

- "There can't be a crisis today—my schedule is already full."
- "Of all the things I've lost, I miss my mind the most."
- "Is it time for *your* medication or *mine*?"
- "Oh-h-h! You meant you want it in a *real* minute?? I thought you meant a *nurse's* minute!"

Last important point here: After using a humorous response, you should then address the problem at hand. The idea isn't to get the other person laughing so hard that you can escape unnoticed [although that might come in handy for some *really* desperate situations!]. You're just trying to decrease the tension at hand so leveler heads can prevail.

———————

(Don't BELIEVE me??) . . .
Here's What *WebMD* Says About Humor & Health

Whatever you're doing right now, stop and find something that makes you laugh. Sure, laughter can help you forget about your troubles, but it also can help your body heal. That's right. Laughter can help your body heal.

Your brain talks to your body

You probably already know that your brain is in charge of things like what you think about and your ability to walk, talk, breathe, and move. But did you know that your brain also produces chemicals that affect everything from how fast your heart beats to how well you fight off disease?

Thanks to something called the mind-body connection, the simple act of laughing can tell your brain to produce chemicals that:

- Lower your risk for heart attacks.

- Increase your blood circulation.

- Help your heart work better and pump more evenly.

- Boost your body's immune system to help you fight off infection.

- Increase your deep breathing, which relaxes your muscles, gives you more energy, and lowers your stress.

- Scientific research backs this up: The more you laugh, the better you'll feel and the healthier you'll be.

    Give it a try.

[http://www.webmd.com/balance/tc/healing-through-humor-topic-overview]

[STILL Don't believe me??] . . .

Check-Out This Humor Research
in the *American Journal of Nursing*

When I wrote my masters thesis on humor and healthcare in the early 1990s [when I was 8 years old], I had to fight to have this topic taken seriously; and there was little solid research to be found. But things have changed in the last 20 years. Here is just a sampling of research in the peer-reviewed *AJN*—the *American Journal of Nursing:*

Is Laughter the Best Medicine?
Pasero, Christine L.; Smith, Nancy; Oliver, Nancy
AJN, American Journal of Nursing. 98(12):12,14, December 1998.
Hospitals and long-term care facilities now utilize humor . . .

Laughter is the Best Medicine: And it's a great adjunct in the treatment of patients with cancer
Pattillo, Charlene Gayle Story; Itano, Joanne
AJN, American Journal of Nursing. 101:40-43, April 2001.
The courage to laugh: humor, hope, and healing in the face of death and dying . . .

Lighten Up!
Starr, Carolina
AJN, American Journal of Nursing. 109(2):72AAA-72BBB, February 2009.
doi: 10.1097/01.NAJ.0000345445.54767.3a
Pain was decreased in subjects exposed simultaneously to humor and . . .

Nursing: A Stand-Up Routine: Smile—the life you save may be your own
Schwarz, Thomas
AJN, American Journal of Nursing. 105:13, 2005.
Look for a mate with a sense of humor. Beauty, wealth—all the initial interests eventually fade . . .

The Power of Play and Laughter
Ekegren, Kathryn
AJN, American Journal of Nursing. 97(11):27-29, November 1997.
A unique sense of humor is a talent . . .

(Excerpts from *U.S. News & World Report*)*

10 Tips to Lighten Up & Laugh

You're never too grown-up to laugh like a kid

by Laura McMullen

Look for humor. "Every day, make a conscious effort to seek humor," Buxman says. Take a two-minute break at the office to watch a video of laughing babies (or whatever your comedy fix is), she says. Record a TV show that makes you laugh. Read the newspaper and look for goofy headlines worthy of Jay Leno's mailbag. "Start looking at the world through that lens of humor," she says. "And you'll be amazed at what you find." Keep a journal of all these little things that make you laugh, Buxman adds, so when you're feeling blue, you have a quick guide for perking up.

Embrace positive laughter. "[Humor] can be a tool that you use positively, but it can also be a weapon," Buxman says. Anyone who's been the butt of a joke, a target of bullies or the recipient of ill-willed sarcasm knows that there's a major difference between laughing with others and being laughed at. As the saying goes, "The richest laugh is at no one's expense."

Don't worry about being funny. "There's a difference between being funny and having a sense of humor," Buxman says. No need to prepare an opening monologue, or to invest in a 12-pack of clown noses. It's OK if you're not the next

Louis CK. Relax, and focus on enjoying and sharing laughs, rather than creating them.

Know your sense of humor. "Sense of humor is very personalized," says Buxman, who's partial to the "Big Bang Theory." But you may laugh at "Girls," or cat videos, or Tyler Perry movies, David Sedaris books or improv shows. Instead of thinking: "Why does everyone think this is funny?" or "I don't get it," figure out what kind of humor does make you howl and schedule time to enjoy it.

[The entire aarticle can be found at *U.S. News & World Report.* April 1, 2013. http://health.usnews.com/health-news/health-wellness/articles/2013/04/01/10-tips-to-lighten-up-and-laugh]

All told, humor really *is* good medicine! It benefits you phsysiologically, psychologically, socially, and it can improve your communications. So don't wait for funny stuff to just *happen* to you . . . Try using humor *intentionally*. You'll reap more benefits that way. Yes, yes, I know that chocolate provides lots of benefits, too. But humor is sweet, too—and it has a lot fewer calories.

"Caring is part of the art of nursing.
Humor is part of the art of caring."

~ KARYN BUXMAN, RN, NEUROHUMORIST

Chapter 3
Humor: The Good, the Bad, and the Ugly

Laughing WITH or Laughing AT?

Wile the U.S. Constitution assures us that "all men are created equal," that venerated document is completely mute on the subject of humor. [John Adams didn't have much of a sense of humor. Apparently, he left that to Benjamin Franklin.]

The Bill of Rights, however, *does* provide for freedom of speech. And this, my fellow funny nurses, is just the opening we're looking for! The following is a paraphrasing of the First Amendment. [Disclaimer: Not intended as legal advice!]

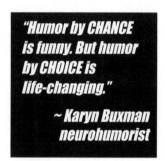

Freedom of speech is the political right to communicate one's opinions and ideas. So this means that if, in a U.S. citizen's opinion, a knock-knock joke about cardiac surgeons is funny, then he or she is allowed to tell it. And, if—in, say, a nurse's opinion—this joke *(Q: How many doctors does it take to change a light bulb? A: Nobody knows. They all expect the nurses to do it!)* cracks-up the nursing staff, then we are allowed to tell/text/blog/share it!

Now, just because we are allowed to *express* humor, does *not* mean that all humor is appropriate, helpful, or healthy.

There are many types of humor, and some kinds of humor are healthier than others. Some kinds of humor make you feel good. And, there are other kinds of humor that can make you feel bad.

Take sarcasm for instance. Personally, I'm a real fan of sarcasm—and chances are that many of the people you work with are, too. In the right setting with the right people, it can be appreciated (see section below on Bond, Environment and Timing). However, some researchers have classified sarcasm as a form of aggressive behavior. It's easy for sarcasm to cross the line into bullying or abusive behavior. (The Greek origin of the word sarcasm, sarkasmós, means "to tear the flesh.") [Ouch!]

If you've ever been sniped with a sarcastic remark, you may feel like you were missing a bit of hide. There are a number of ways to respond to aggressive sarcasm, ranging from simply saying "Really??" to taking the commenter aside to let him or her know they're not all that funny. Ignoring remarks that bother you may *seem* like an effective coping strategy, but the truth is that sarcasm may lead to increased levels of anger and frustration. Establishing and maintaining boundaries regarding the types of humor people can use with you is a vital part of self-care.

Understanding the TYPES of Humor

Humor comes in a number of flavors. There's *constructive* humor—the light, upbeat type of humor that builds people up. (A side benefit is that it builds *you* up, too!) And then there's *destructive* humor, which is a more negative type of humor, where we find the laughs at other people's expense. Wise to avoid!

Which is which? If you would feel ashamed if

someone you respect heard the joke you just told, it's likely negative humor. If someone you didn't like told you the joke, would you find yourself offended or incensed? Negative humor.

It's a matter of laughing genuinely *with* someone versus laughing *at* someone. It's always healthier to laugh *with* others than to laugh *at* them. Occasionally you may find yourself in the predicament of not being able to help yourself from laughing at someone. Here's a line that may keep you out of trouble: "I'm sorry that I'm laughing. It reminds me of the time I (fill-in-the- blank)." Now you've turned the laughter back on yourself instead of onto the other person. Generally a wise thing to do.

To build bonds and strengthen relationships among your team, you want to practice humor that makes others feel safe. One technique that usually works well is self-deprecating humor—making fun of yourself. No one will be offended, and it will actually show people that your self-esteem is strong enough to withstand being teased. Self-deprecating humor can actually increase other people's opinion of you!

A Word (or 872) about "Sick" Humor

One kind of humor that falls into the gray zone is "sick humor." When tragedy and death cloud our lives, they darken our humor as well. Anyone who has to

deal with issues that are tragic or unfair is a great can-
didate for sick humor (also known as dark humor, gal-
lows humor, or black humor).

Guess where nurses fall on this scale?? People who
know first-hand the harsh realities of healthcare are
among the world's biggest fans of sick humor. (Our
colleagues in dealing first-hand with human tragedy
and suffering include police officers, firefighters and
soldiers. On behalf of your nurse cousins, I salute
you!) That being said, I must confess that most nurses
are special fans of humor featuring body fluids, death
and dismembership. [Please don't tell our mothers!]

"All bleeding stops . . . eventually."
~ ANN NONYMOUS

Anyone who deals with traumatic situations is likely to count on some type of "sick humor" to help
them keep their balance amid difficult situations. For
example, police officers, fire fighters and soldiers all
have their own styles of dark humor that helps them
get by, and also bonds them to one another. It's a special brand of humor that is not meant for outsiders.
And that makes sense, because if you've never experienced what *they* have, you're not really a member of
their "tribe."

Any kind of humor that makes you laugh, whether
it's sick or not, is going to relieve some of your stress.

It may not, however, do much for the stress of the people *around* you! Those who share your pain and experiences as a nurse will "get it." Those who don't, won't. That's just the way it is.

Risky Business (and the B.E.T. Method)

Have you ever tried to be funny and put your foot in your mouth? [I certainly have!] There's almost always some degree of risk involved when you use humor. My purpose in sharing these insights is to help you push the cost/benefit ratio into the plus column. Here are three ways to take some of the risk out of the risky business of humor, and make your humor a safe B.E.T. (B stands for "Bond"; E stands for "Environment"; and T stands for "Timing.")

B = Bond

The Bond represents those places in which you have a point of commonality with the people you're about to share your humor with. How are you connected? Are they work colleagues? Are they neighbors? High school pals? Drinking buddies? If you have a close relationship with your listeners, you'll definitely know what will make them laugh. But if your relationship is newer or more casual, then you won't be on such firm ground.

Use some common sense here. Consider the people you're with at the time. Are they the type of people who get offended easily? If so, you'll want to hold back on some types of humor. On the other hand, if you're with a bunch of George Carlin fans, you know that your humor can be sharper.

The longer you've known the people, and the better your relationship is with them, the safer your humor will be. If you've shared some gross-out humor with your long-time nurse pal, she's probably going to overlook the ickiness, not be offended, and will probably laugh heartily. However, if it's someone you've known for only a short time (a patient, for instance), or have only known casually (the equipment rep who shows up once a year), you may want to edit some of your humor before sharing it with them.

E = Environment

Being aware of the environment also helps determine if humor is appropriate. There's a saying that, "There's a time and a place for everything," and environment is all about the place. As nurses, we have to make sure that our use of humor doesn't have a negative impact on the healthcare environment. This can be a balancing act: You want to use humor enough that the patients feel more relaxed, but not so much humor that they question your professionalism or skill.

Anyone who *hears* your humor, *sees* your humor, or *experiences* your humor is part of your audience, whether you mean for them to be or not. The patient who appears to be safely off in dreamland might actually be hearing every single word you say. An ounce of caution is worth an entire afternoon of explaining and apologizing!

T = Timing

You can have the right audience, in the right setting, and use humor—only to have it fall flat. Timing is perhaps the most difficult element to master when using humor. Have you ever heard people say, "Too soon!" to jokes about unfortunate events? They're not ready to laugh about the situation yet.

How can you tell if the timing is right? How much time must elapse before an event can be funny? To be able to laugh at an experience, you need to be able to emotionally detach from it. It has to be possible for you to look at the circumstances without re-experiencing the emotional response you had when the event occurred.

That process of detaching can take time. It's not an instant process—nor should it be! As complete human beings, we experience a wide range of emotions in response to life events. Anger, frustration, upset, and embarrassment all have their role to play. At the peak of a crisis things simply ain't that funny. But we learn from our life experiences (eventually!), and they help us grow.

After we've learned those lessons, it's time to laugh. Have you ever found yourself saying, "Someday I'm going to laugh about this"? One option that people rarely consider is to consciously choose to shorten that timeframe. It *is* possible!

Any accident or mishap has a lot of potential to be Very Not Funny. But *sometimes* there *is* laughter to be found, at least according to one colleague who told me about an experience as a new nurse:

> "My patient was rolled over on his side; I had just finished giving him an enema. Then without thinking, I bent over to pick up some linen that had fallen to the floor—when *Bam!*—the patient had an explosive reaction to the enema—right in my face."
>
> Seeing my horrified expression, my friend laughed and said, "Oh, it was no big deal . . . I had my mouth shut!"

Some people can distance themselves immediately. They can laugh at their own mistakes—whether it's driving out of the parking lot with a sack of groceries on the roof of the car, or saying something dumb in a meeting.

But other people need more time to process their reactions and emotions. When some people make a mistake, they berate themselves harshly. And as long as they are emotionally attached to the painful event, they will not find it funny.

> *Laughter lightens one's mood.*
>
> *Humor supports intimacy.*
>
> *Frivolity reduces fear.*

And then there are those folks who will just *never* see the situation as funny. And that's okay, too. None of us have the right to force our own coping style—or humor style—on anyone else.

Effective stress management involves practicing emotionally detaching from painful events, searching instead for the humor those moments contain. It isn't always easy, but with practice you'll find that you've developed the "Humor Habit."

WHEN to Use Humor

Sometimes it is difficult to tell whether humor is appropriate in a given situation. Many times, we're so worried about whether laughing is really the right thing to do at any particular moment, that we censor ourselves, stopping ourselves from using humor.

This is the "When in doubt, leave it out" approach. This is undoubtedly the *safest* option. Use it *too* often, however, and you may leave yourself unable to capitalize on some of the many benefits of humor.

It's also important to remember to refrain from using humor during moments of crisis, or when it's vitally important that communication be clear and concise. Humor often works by distracting the attention, and there are times when distraction is a Very Bad Idea.

Before using humor, do a quick mental "time-out":

- What is my *connection* with the audience?
- Is this the right *setting* for this type of humor?
- Is this the right *time* to use humor?

The SAFEST Form of Humor

When in doubt about what kind of humor to use with others, use self-effacing humor (making fun of yourself). Sharing a funny story about yourself shows self-confidence and yet also shows vulnerability.

People find this kind of humor totally non-threatening, and they may feel secure enough to share their own humor back with you.

Note 1: With self-effacing humor, it's best to focus on the dopey thing you *did*, rather than on the dopey person you *are*!

Note 2: Using self-effacing humor requires self-confidence and a strong sense of who you really are.

"Laugh at your actions, not at who you are.
It's safer to admit that you MADE a mistake
than to admit that you ARE a mistake."

~ TERRY PAULSON, PhD

My friend and humor colleague, Linda MacNeal, refers to self-deprecating humor as "Human Humor," saying that she values the ability to laugh at the fact she's only human. This is a really healthy framework to use when we choose to poke fun at our own failings and foibles.

Remember this: You are *somebody*. Somebody who can be strong enough and confident enough to poke fun at yourself. Remember this, too: People who never use self-deprecating humor are not as confident and strong as they would like you to believe!

"I always wanted to be somebody . . . but now I realize I should have been more specific."
~ LILY TOMLIN

Self-deprecating humor is a powerful technique to help you deal with a stressful career, not to mention your everyday life.

Seriously. The world does *enough* to tear us down. We don't have to do it to ourselves.

"Some days you need tools. Other days you need weapons. But you need your sense of humor every day."

~ MELODIE CHENEVERT, RN

Chapter 4
Laughter IS the Best Medicine: Humor and Your Patients

Being a nurse is hard—but being a patient is even harder.

Sometimes that's difficult to remember. A day full of frequent fliers, drug seekers, and patients who are sure they'd be fine if you'd just "Get Dr. House, already!" can leave you feeling a little short in the empathy department.

That's understandable, and it helps to acknowledge that it happens. Many of the situations we encounter are frustrating. But we can't *stay* in that frustrated mindset without negatively affecting patient care.

Rick Segel, an expert in workplace behavior, has identified a phenomenon called "Last Customer Residue" in which the interaction with an unpleasant customer spills over (and often ruins!) the interaction that a salesperson has with his or her *next* customer. In much the same way, our experience with the *last* patient influences our interaction with the *next* patient. And that's not necessarily a good thing.

Walking a Mile in Someone Else's Crocs: Understanding Patients

To stop the cycle of negativity in its tracks, it helps to remember that 99.9% of the time, our patients would rather be anywhere else on the planet. Not many people wake up in the morning saying, "Hurray! I get to have open heart surgery today!" Few folks spend their days hoping against hope that they'll develop rheumatoid arthritis. No one's fondest hope is that they someday get to experience COPD.

Our patients are our patients because they're dealing with medical *problems*. When we see people, they're not necessarily having their best day ever. And that's before we factor in whatever *other* stressors those patients are facing—family, financial, personal, social or professional.

And don't forget that your patients may have just

spent a lot of time waiting impatiently in the waiting room—with other sick, injured, bored or scared people.

As nurses, we're very comfortable spending time in the medical setting. We spend every day surrounded by physicians, diagnostic equipment, IV bags and sick people. This isn't true for our patients, who can find these sights unfamiliar, upsetting, or just plain frightening. And even the language we use everyday is not familiar to them, and this can create confusion.

"When I was a naïve CNA," Brenda Jahnke, MSN, RN, CSN, said, "I once told a patient that I was there to take his vitals. He clasped his hands over his private parts and replied, "Honey, I don't have *much*—and you can't take it!"

I was dumbfounded as to why he said that until . . . then we both laughed."

Humor fights frustration.

Humor helps people support others.

Humor provides perspective.

When we remember that our patients are confused, stressed, and maybe even scared, it makes us better nurses. When we can use humor to help them transition into a calmer, less anxious emotional state, everyone benefits. Patient outcomes are better, and our interactions with them are more positive and productive. This makes our work more satisfying, and as a result, we're happier people. [And, of course, it's all about *us*, isn't it? Ha!]

A lot of good can come from a little laughter.

8 Humor Strategies to Help Your Patients

1. Decrease Fear by Increasing Frivolity

We see the best patient outcomes from patients who come to us in a calm, centered emotional state. Ideally, they'll be fully informed about what's going to happen, including the benefits they'll get from the procedure, and some idea of what the healing process will be like. Patients should be free from anxiety, stress, and fear.

Now raise your hand if you've ever had a patient like that. Don't feel bad if you can't. These types of patients are few and far between! None of us live in an ideal world. Our patients come to us more than a little anxious.

It is important to make sure that your patients really do understand the situation at hand. Again, if you an get your patients to laugh, you can get them to listen—and they'll be better able to comprehend your message.

> Laurie worked with patients with dia-
> betes and heart disease, many of whom
> were non-compliant. Then one day, she
> purchased a funny prop to help convey
> the importance of diet: A rubber blob of
> imitation human fat, the size of a soccer
> ball!
>
> When a patient seemed to be losing
> interest, or not grasping the importance
> of what she was saying, she would pull
> out the blob of fat and plop it into the
> patient's outstretched hands. After the
> inevitable gasp, the patient would laugh
> and then recognize Laurie's point.

Having your patients explain to you, in their own words, the procedure they're going to have, can be a source of mirth and delight for both of you. One older gentleman, awaiting an orchiectomy, proudly reported that the doctor was going to change him "from a rooster into a hen!"

These conversations can relieve some of the tension the patient is experiencing—and it can also open the door to larger conversations. That particular patient had some concerns about his future sex life that had been weighing heavily on his mind. Because he was able to laugh about the situation with the nurse first, he felt safe enough in the clinical environment to bring up his worries.

2. Lower Patients' Stress with Delight & Diversion

Murphy's Law of Patientology: "The more freaked out and afraid a patient is, the longer he or she will have to wait to see the doctor."

Anticipation is a powerful force. Research conducted by Dr. Lee Berk, a leading psychoneuroimmunologist, has found that looking forward to a fun event (watching a movie, going out to dinner, going on vacation) can have nearly as many health benefits as enjoying the event itself. Negative anticipation (a state of being fearful in advance—dreading what is to come) has the opposite effect. (Note: These health benefits are not broad guesses. They arespecific, measurable positive changes in body systems such as respiratory, musculo-skeletal and immune.)

There is no environment on earth more prone to negative anticipation than the waiting room in a hospital or clinic! Spend half an hour among your soon-to-be patients, and you'll quickly pick-up on the fearful, negative vibe. You'll meet the gal who's waiting to see the gastroenterologist—and you'll learn about the inner workings of her bowels, in excruciating detail. You'll meet the sweaty guy suffering from the disease-of-the-week. You'll read the latest news, about the Apollo moon landing, in a four-decades-old edition of *National Geographic*. You'll discover that there's really not much to do in the waiting room except sit there and dwell on what's about to happen to you, and the many ways it could all go wrong.

It's easy to see why patients' imaginations are likely to run amok creating all kinds of negative scenarios. Maybe the doctor will have horrible news. Maybe you'll need surgery. Maybe you'll need surgery *immediately*. Maybe your condition is so bad that the doctor will have to operate on you right there on the waiting room coffee table!

> *Recent studies show that people who actively use humor have lower levels of markers for inflammation (C-reactive proteins and cytokines) which lead to atherosclerosis and cardiovascular disease.*

You can see how this doesn't necessarily result in a calm and emotionally centered patient.

How might you help your patients combat their negative mindset? With delight and diversion, of course! These two humor strategies are powerful tools for countering negative anticipation. Humor delights and distracts people, and improves their mental outlook.

One way to create delight and diversion is to make the waiting area genuinely patient-friendly. I have vis-

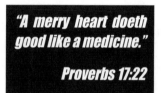

ited several facilities that have done a great job making that environment more cheerful and upbeat. Pastel-colored walls are more soothing than gun metal grey. Fun and funny posters are more uplifting than dime store prints of sad clowns.

Two warnings regarding TVs in waiting rooms: First, soap operas ain't funny. And second, TVs tuned to the news are, essentially, stress-creating machines.

One clinic I visited keeps a basket of comic strips in the waiting room. Staff members bring in their favorites. One of the nurses suggested that they lamiate copies of the comics, and invite patients to take home their favorite. Much to the surprise and delight of the staff, patients began bringing in comics to contribute to the basket! And here's what's especially noteworthy about this idea: Something that was begun "Just for fun" ended up being something that entertained and distracted patients while they were waiting for their appointments. [I *told* you that humor works wonders!]

Another strategy is to encourage patients to distract themselves. As a nurse, you can provide this encouragement directly . . . "Just be careful how you do it!" says Veronica Thomas, RN, Director of Nursing for Northeast Missouri Ambulatory Surgery Center:

> We discovered that our pediatric patients did much better if they had something fun to do while they were waiting for their procedure. So we got some handheld video games—Gameboys—for the kids to play with. They loved them. This was when Gameboys were fairly new and very cool.
>
> One of our nurses, who wasn't very familiar with kids' toys, brings in a peds patient. Then, remembering our new protocol involving the new Gameboys, she turns to the little guy and says, "While you're waiting, would you like me to get you a—um—a—a *Playboy*?"

[Oops!]

3. Listen Beyond the Laughter

Humor has many important roles to play in the healing process. One of the most important occurs when patients use jokes and laughter as a way to address topics that they're not comfortable speaking about directly. When patients use humor, it's often a good sign that they're processing the many complex feelings that go along with their situation.

"You can give it to me straight, Doc: Will I be able to play the piano after this?"

"Sure!"

"Well, that's great! I've never even had a lesson!"

What seems like a simple joke can be a sign that there are concerns and questions that need to be addressed—preferably before the treatment progresses any further.

The American Medical Association reports that 73% of all patients worry about their physician making a mistake. People are using the internet to double-check what they've been told about their diagnosis and treatment options—and let's just say that not every website out there is as credible as WebMD. It has been found that knowledgable patients have more confidence in their treatment, and this can have a huge impact on their subsequent experiences.

And with that in mind, remember that our patients

are subject to cultural forces and social pressures that discourage them from directly questioning authority figures. A patient who would never question a doctor face-to-face may easily use Facebook to tell the world that her doctor is a quack. She may, however, use humor to tell her nurse. Using humor—even dark, borderline, "inappropriate" humor—gives people a safe way to talk about things that are troubling them.

As professional caregivers we must, of course, maintain appropriate standards for the therapeutic environment—and it is important for us to focus on what's actually being communicated. With this in mind, it's important that we learn to listen beyond the laughter.

When we do that, we create opportunities to identify points of need and anxiety that we can actually remedy. Sometimes it's as simple as conveying accurate information or clarifying medical terminology. This can provide tremendous peace of mind for patients.

In other instances, we may not have any answers— but we can still be there to listen and provide compassionate support.

4. Equip Yourself for Life's Embarrassing Moments

I've conducted extensive research, delving deeply into the medical literature in order to confirm what nurses have long suspected: Embarrassment is not, in fact, a fatal condition.

Good luck trying to get your patients to believe that! There's a lot that happens in healthcare that can provoke feelings of embarrassment—even extreme mortification! For many people, being partially undressed in front of others is very uncomfortable. The stylish exam gowns are only the tip of the iceberg. Who can forget those precious post-operative moments when it's time to get rid of excessive internal gas?

It's important to understand that embarrassment is a very visceral reaction. Intellectually, patients understand that the body has ways to eliminate the build-up of gas. They know the process is natural and they may even accept that it is necessary. But that intellectual knowledge pales against the feelings of humiliation that can come with passing gas where other people can hear (and smell!) it.

As nurses, we can use humor to show these patients that they're not alone. One way to do this is by sharing our own embarrassing experiences. When one's face is red, it helps a lot to know that someone else has been in a similar situation—and survived the experience . . . and could laugh about it later!

Flatulence is not the only source of embarrassment in a healthcare setting. When I was teaching nursing, I loved to share this story about my experience working as a circulating nurse:

> One morning, while I was hurrying down the hallway to circulate for a C-section, I saw a tall, young man in scrubs looking somewhat lost. "Must be the soon-to-be father," I thought. Out loud I asked, "Are you looking for the C-section?"
>
> He nodded uncertainly.
>
> I said, "Well, you can't go into the operating room without a mask! Follow me."
>
> I took him by the elbow, and led him—gently-but-firmly—over to the scrub sink, where I showed him the proper way to wash his hands. I then handed him a mask. "You take these two strings and tie them like *this* . . ." I demonstrated, " . . . and you take these two strings and tie them—like *so*!"
>
> The man nodded slowly, then replied, "Thank you. But I prefer to tie mine like *this*." He then extended his hand to me. "I'm the new pediatrician, Dr. McHardy."

I smiled back, shook his hand enthusias-
tically, and without hesitation said,
"Welcome! I'm *Nancy Roberts*, the OR
supervisor."

It was two weeks before he discovered
that I'm not Nancy Roberts!"

Sometimes—often when you least expect it—life
provides you with exactly the embarrassing moment
your patients need to get over their own feelings of
humiliation. One nurse shared:

I had a patient who, due to her faith community, was a very modest woman. And
we were doing our best to respect that,
and she was doing her best to go along
with what needed to be done, but it was
clearly very uncomfortable for her.

Luckily, I am the World's Clumsiest
Nurse. I'm in there, working on the IV,
and one wrong move and you guessed
it—saline shower, head to toe, I'm
soaked. Luckily we don't wear white on
my unit—but you could still see way
more of me than I was comfortable with!

My patient burst out laughing. "Now
we're even!" she said. "You see me, I see

you!" I couldn't help but laugh along. That moment changed things for us. It made it a little easier for us to do what had to be done.

[This reminds me of the adage "Never Let Them See You Sweat." Apparently, it is *also* true that "Dripping Saline All Over The Place Works Wonders."]

5. Get Them Laughing, Get Them Learning!

This year, there will be approximately 53,000 tonsillectomies performed in the US. This means that there will be more than 53,000 times that patients will receive detailed instructions about the best way to conduct themselves in order to effect a speedy and complete recovery.

Let's be real here: These instructions aren't brain surgery [or even rocket science!]. "Don't pick up heavy objects, stick to clear fluids for a while, and monitor for fever or signs of infection." There's nothing on this list that should confuse anyone. This is simple stuff.

Yet I guarantee you that in an emergency room somewhere near you, a post-tonsillectomy patient is presenting, right this very minute, with excruciating pain. It will turn out, upon investigation, that Cool Ranch Doritos are not, in fact, a clear liquid.

How in the world does this happen? What's going wrong here? Undergoing surgery can be scary and overwhelming. Patients who are anxious often develop a type of tunnel vision, where they can only see what they need to see in order to get out of the surgery center as quickly as possible. They're so focused on "getting out of Dodge," and back home, that any possible distraction—even something as helpful as patient education—becomes meaningless background noise to them.

> "The ability to laugh—either naturally or as a learned behavior—may have important implications in societies such as the U.S. where heart disease remains the number one killer."
>
> ~ Dr. Michael Miller

Not all patients have surgery, but almost all patients need some kind of education. The specific information on how to take one's medicine, or follow a heart-healthy diet, or use an inhaler when they feel an asthma attack coming on: All of this stuff is vital information that our patients have an alarming tendency to tune out.

This is where humor helps. Humor is a disruptive force—[that's why the teacher doesn't love the Class Clown]—and this disruptive force can be harnessed to help our patients move from that single-minded focus of "I-want-to-go-home! I-want-to-go-home!" to a place where they can be open-to and aware-of the information they'll need to heal properly.

Let's say we're talking about recovery times. We can share the straightforward facts, or, in those instances where it appears that the patient may not actually be paying attention, try using humor to get through. Here's a story that I've used in that situation:

> Two little boys were in a hospital, about to go in for surgery. The first boy asked the second, "What are you in here for?" The second boy said he was going to have his tonsils out. The first boy comforted the second, explaining that it wasn't so bad: "A bit of a sore throat, and lots of ice cream! And you'll be playing really soon!"

> The second boy then asked what his new buddy was in for. The first boy replied that he was getting circumcised. The second boy shook his head sadly and said, "Oh no! I had a circumcision when I was a baby, and I couldn't walk for a year!"

It takes most patients a moment to get it—and the "Ah-ha! moment" shifts their awareness. They become more fully present in the moment, and that means more attention paid to post-op instructions—and, all things being equal, fewer Cool Ranch Doritos.

Humor is not a magic bullet. You won't get every patient to pay attention by making them laugh. But for the ones who stop, and listen, and laugh, there's a greater chance they're going to remember and comply with instructions. And that leads directly to better patient outcomes.

6. Use High-Touch, Not Just High-Tech

Medicine is a science *and* an art—and it's often the *art* part that leaves many doctors stymied. Humor can play a role in closing the communication gap that often crops up between the technically-expert, focused clinical team, and the very, very human patient.

> Our patient satisfaction surveys had revealed that while our standard of care was excellent, patients felt the whole process was too mechanical and impersonal. They wanted more direct interaction with the physician. Specifically, they wanted the doctors to touch them. It didn't matter if the doctor could diagnose them simply by reading their x-ray; there was something about physical contact that made them feel better cared-for.

We tried to communicate this to one of our docs—a great orthopedic surgeon, but not a touchy-feely kind of guy. He listened attentively, and said he'd try to do better. So in comes the next patient, a little old lady who needed surgery on her elbow. She's a fiesty gal, and a bit on the plump side.

The doctor is reading the x-ray while reaching under the blanket and palpating the complaint area—when the woman looks him straight in the eye and says, "Honey, I'm not going to stop you . . . But if you think that's my elbow, you're sadly mistaken!"

7. Empower Your Patients

Why are our patients anxious and stressed-out? Part of the reason is that participating in the health-care system today requires surrendering a significant amount of control—far more than we do at most other times in our lives. Wearing a revealing gown, being without one's phone or computer (often more stressful than the surgery itself!), or being on one's own without family or friends around can be an over-whelming experience.

One of the ways patients try to deal with this (and enjoy better outcomes) is by being vigilant about their care. They want to be informed. The more they know about what's going on, the more they feel in control of the situation.

We should never forget that *humor is power*. One of the ways people use humor is to give themselves back some of the power they feel they've lost. To do this, they sometimes tease or poke gentle fun at the people who surround them.

Sometimes that means they're teasing *you* . . .

> I had a friend, Pat, who was doing home health visits on patients receiving chemotherapy at home. Pat was seeing a man who was going to receive 5FU for the first time, so she spent most of the visit teaching him about the procedure, the pump, and the drug. She went over some of the side effects of the chemo, which included hair loss. She completed her visit and said she would be back tomorrow.
>
> The next day Pat rang the doorbell and was greeting by the patient's anxious-looking wife. She said, "You are *not* going to believe this!" She led Pat into the living room . . . where she stopped dead in her tracks.

> Her patient was *completely* bald. He looked at her and said, "I know you said I might lose *some* of my hair—but *all* of it?!" Pat just stood there, mouth open, not knowing what to say . . . when all of a sudden the man and his wife burst out laughing.
>
> Pat was perplexed and worried—until her patient held up a furry object . . . which turned out to be his toupè!

Humor is *also* helpful to patients of all ages. AARP recognizes the power of humor in the healing process. AARP's blog, "Humor Therapy" includes these pieces: "Days of Laughter, Days of Grief"—about the role of humor in one man's battle with colon cancer; and "Humor Therapy Helps Dementia Patients"—about how humor can improve the quality of life for those suffering from dementia.

[http://blog.aarp.org/tag/humor-therapy/]

8. Build Resiliency with Humor

As nurses, we don't treat symptoms. We don't cure diseases. Our patients are far more than their diagnosis or CPT code: *They're people*, complete and whole, who come to us with far more than their immediate medical needs. How many times have you seen patients who have really serious health problems— only to discover that those issues pale in comparison to what they're facing in their romantic relationship, family life or workplace?

By modeling the therapeutic use of humor, we're providing patients with a tool they can use to address stressors in every sphere of their lives. Laughter's benefits are universally applicable. The emotional relief that comes from enjoying humor allows us to build the resiliency we need to keep facing down life's biggest challenges.

> *Humor rewards and recognizes.*
>
> *Humor levels social hierarchies.*
>
> *Humor encourages openness.*

"Do I love coming here every other day for dialysis? No, I don't," Tom R. said. "But I love the fact that one of the ladies who works here is going to make me laugh. I always leave with a smile on my face. I think *that* does more to keep me going than anything else."

One way to get your patients laughing is to give them a peek behind the scenes. People love to imagine

that they're in their very own episode of *Scrubs*...
Little do they realize that real life in the hospital can be
even funnier:

The Top Ten Worst Visitors—Ever!

10. The man who snuck his three cats into the
    hospital to visit his asthmatic wife.
9. The visitor who ate all his father's food, then
    rang the nurse to say that the patient was still
    hungry and needed another meal.
8. The obstinate six-year-old who kept
    changing Grandpa's TV from the Golf
    Channel to *SpongeBob SquarePants*.
7. The son who emptied his mother's
    colostomy bag into the wastebasket at the
    nurse's station.
6. The male visitor who fell asleep in the
    patient's bed while she was in the bathroom.
5. The wife who discontinued her husband's
    CVP line herself, because "John likes to sleep
    on his right side."
4. The 80-year-old daughter of the 98-year-old
    man, who kept drinking her father's
    continuous IV fluids when she got thirsty.
3. The children of one patient who used
    their mother's portable IPPB machine as a
    scooter in the hallway.

2. The husband who kept sneaking in choco-
    lates for his newly diagnosed diabetic wife.
    The jig was up when he hid them under her
    roommate's bed—and the whole room
    became infested with cockroaches.

1. The man who never actually visited his
    brother, but called dozens of times, round-
    the-clock, day-after-day to criticize the
    nurses, the doctors, the food, and the lack
    of parking!

Patients are wonderful. Patients are aggravating.
Patients are a challenge. Patients give us purpose. And
patients deserve our best. The best of our talents, or
expertise, our skills, our compassion . . . and our sense
of humor.

*"Nothing is quite as funny
as the unintentional humor of reality."*

~ STEVE ALLEN

"Our bodies are helped to heal by engaging in activities that bring us joy and fulfillment.

Play is mandatory, it is not elective."

~ O. CARL SIMONTON, MD

Chapter 5
It Takes a Village:
Humor & Your Healthcare Team

Over the years, I've spoken to thousands of nurses. From the most freshly graduated student nurses to the extra experienced types, we all have one thing in common: Our fellow nurses. Our colleagues are our greatest resource and inspiration. And yet, it's these same colleagues and co-workers who can be our greatest source of stress and frustration.

The high-pressure, intense environment we function in, coupled with the demanding work we do, can bring out the best in all of us. It can also bring out the worst.

In a perfect world, we could count on having positive professional relationships with everyone we work with. Respect would come standard, and no one would ever dump their frustration and anger on the nearest nurse.

But we don't live in a perfect world. Interpersonal relations can be the toughest part of the workplace. Abrasive doctors, hostile colleagues, administrators who are constantly urging that a higher standard of care be provided with fewer resources. Does any of this sound familiar?

"Nursing would be a dream job—
if it weren't for the doctors!"

~ GERHARD KOCKER, SWISS HEALTH-ECONOMIST

These aren't situations that can be ignored. The nursing profession deserves more. Each one of us, as an individual nurse endowed with personal dignity and hard-earned professional skills, deserves more.

Humor can help us get what we deserve. Sociologists suggest that part of the reason humor is such a natural, universal part of the human experience is that laughter functions as a social lubricant.

Laughing makes relationships work better—so much so that we sometimes laugh even when nothing is funny! University of Maryland Professor Robert

Provine found evidence that a primary purpose of laughter is to serve as a social signal, indicating that someone is friendly, good natured, and non-threatening. In other words, laughter is not always an indication that there's observable humor present.

Laughter is also a way to communicate social messages to each other, conveying whether behavior is acceptable or not. When we laugh at a situation, we're giving a tacit approval of the behavior being displayed. Sometimes this is a good thing, while other times it's problematical. Part of using humor therapeutically is developing the ability to recognize when our use of humor is healthy and when it's perpetuating cycles that need to stop.

In this section, we'll be discussing how to do that.

9 Humor Strategies to Support (and Survive) Your Colleagues

1. Create a Safe Space to Process Emotions Through Humor

Have you ever had this experience? . . . You're talking with a family member or a neighbor about your work day, and he or she says, "I know exactly how you feel!"—and you want to scream, *"No, you don't! You didn't feel the joy of a baby's birth! You didn't feel the sorrow of an old man's death! You didn't feel the fear of a dozen confused and frightened patients!"*

But of course you don't scream. You're a professional caregiver. So you smile and nod your head. And you stuff those emotions down—down on top of the previous layers of unprocessed emotions.

Does anyone else see the makings of a powder keg here??

A little therapy might help. A little vacation might help. A little—or a lot—of chocolate might help. But for day-to-day fast relief of nagging emotions—there's nothing like laughter! [Did that sound like an ad?! Hey, if I could bottle laughter like aspirin, I would be a *billionaire!*]

> *Humor creates community.*
>
> *Humor builds history.*
>
> *Humor helps people accept change.*

Whether you're faced with traumatic situations, or just everyday aggravations, humor can help you survive and thrive. Sometimes all you have to do it shift your mindset: You *could* see the screaming doctor as a little boy throwing a tantrum.

Your sense of humor can create a buffer between you and the people and situations that might otherwise overwhelm you or drive you crazy. Your sense of humor is a powerful tool in your toolbox of survival skills. Wield it often!

2. Build a Humor Library: FOR NURSES ONLY!

One quick and simple way to support the humor habit among your team is to build a humor library. No, you don't need to build shelves or buy books! A humor library can be as simple as a binder filled with cartoons, funny stories, and jokes. Leave it in the staff lounge or break room where everyone can enjoy and add to it—with the understanding that while all material is intended for the nurses, it could, at any time, be read by anyone in the building. It's a good idea to keep things family-friendly and positive for that reason.

Your humor library could include books, magazines and funny movies on DVD, as well as cartoons, newspaper clippings and jokes. Online resources, such as invitation-only Facebook groups, are also a great way to share jokes and humor with your team.

I've seen hospital humor libraries that were contained in a box. But don't be afraid to think outside the box! Your humor library could be a bulletin board, a shelf, a binder, a table or an online group!

3. Leveling the Playing Field with Humor

Humor is power. It is so powerful that it can shatter rigid hierarchies! Laughter puts people on a level playing field. And that's very important in healthcare, because our health care system today is still extremely hierarchical.

Every member of the healthcare team has a vital role to play, with specific contributions to make toward the patient's successful outcome. Every member of the healthcare team is a highly trained healthcare professional. However, every member of the healthcare team does not receive the same amount of social recognition or validation for their professional skills—from the general public, or even from each other.

For a number of cultural and social reasons, a hierarchy has emerged over time, with doctors receiving the lion's share of prestige and respect. This hierarchal dynamic pervades healthcare, with each person finding a role to occupy based on position, experience, and gender. A white male neurosurgeon is treated differently than a Latina female CNA—by every single person that each of them encounters throughout the day. [Does that sound Politically Incorrect? So be it. I call 'em as I see 'em.]

Like all hierarchies, things look pretty good from

the top. But if you're lower down on the totem pole, things often aren't so great. Leveling social hierarchies as much as possible enhances team functionality, particularly when that team needs to function in a high-stress environment.

Humor helps to level social hierarchies. When people laugh together over shared experiences, for that moment, they're all on the same level. There is no upper-or-lower, better-or-worse. The surgeon is on the same footing as the scrub nurse. Humor illustrates what we have in common, rather than focusing on those factors that differentiate us from each other.

The following is another True Story from The Karyn Buxman, RN Files. [Proving, once again, that you don't have to make this stuff up!]

> During nursing school one day I was scheduled to follow my orthopedic case study into a lengthy surgery. As I was changing into my scrubs I realized that I had thrown *two left shoes* into my bag. I was smiling when I told my nursing instructor about my little mistake. But I wasn't smiling when he expressed zero empathy, ordered me to don both left shoes, and hurry into surgery!
>
> What followed was the single most

physically uncomfortable day I have experienced in my entire life. I walked like I had a neuromuscular disease!

Later, during my years as a nursing instructor, I loved telling this story to my students. First, because of the laugh it generated. But second, because it allowed my students to connect with me—because my painful experience as a newbie leveled the playing field between professor and students.

4. Boost Morale with Humor

No matter what type of nursing you practice, one thing is certain: There are going to be good days, and there are going to be bad days. Humor can play a vital role in determining how well your team navigates the bad days. Nurses who laugh regularly when things are going well build themselves a set of coping tools they can draw upon to help them during the tough times.

From a fellow nurse . . .

In long-term care, well, it is what it is. Most of our patients won't be going home again. They all have good days and bad days. But most of them are wonderful people! And we all have our favorites.

On our unit, Ramon was our favorites. This little old Italian man was such a sweetheart. He'd tell everyone, *"When I get out of this place, I'm gonna take you home and marry you!"*

When we lost him, it hit us hard. You know it's going to happen, but that doesn't really make it easier. I mean, we were all down in the dumps.

The next week, one of my favorite fellow nurses needed help to transfer one of our larger patients. And so of course I gave her a hand. And when we were done, she looked at me and said, *"When I get out of this place, I'm gonna take you home and marry you!"*

We both laughed so hard we cried. And it caught on. To this day, when one of us does something nice for another, instead of saying, 'Thanks,' we'll say, *"When I get out of this place, I'm gonna take you home and marry you!"* It makes us laugh, and it helps us remember Ramon.

All nurses go through some pretty intense experiences. Trauma cases are inherently stressful.

Sometimes the patients we're pulling for the most don't do very well. There are problems even the most skilled professionals can't fix. Every team experiences sad times, grieving times and healing times. Humor can play a role in easing the transition from grieving to healing.

Laughing after loss is important in a team's journey back to equilibrium.

The key to using humor in these instances is to be subtle and strategic . . .

> One month was particularly hard on our [oncology] unit. First we lost a teenage boy who had been battling leukemia for over a year. A week later, an 8-year-old girl who had become the darling of our unit lost her battle to cancer, as well. And the very next week yet another little boy, a 4-year-old twin, died from complications from his treatment.
>
> We *know* that these things happen on units like ours, but we were just walking around like zombies. The our unit manager started sending out short funny emails. Just a joke or a funny picture, and the subject line was always the same: "When you need a smile today." It was a subtle gesture—and don't get me wrong,

we still cried—but we started laughing again, too. And we needed that.

A little laughter can go a long way. Visual humor, such as cartoons or funny pictures, deliver a lot of bang for the buck. That's because we process imagery differently than we do text or spoken words. The laughter comes faster, and more automatically— bypassing the self-imposed filters we often place on ourselves when we feel sad or depressed. The mood-lifting benefits of laughter are near immediate. Even a little laughter will have some positive effect on team morale.

5. Recognize & Reward with Humor

When was the last time someone told you that you did a good job? When was the last time *you* expressed your admiration to a colleague for the fine work he or she does?

It's important to make the time. There are benefits to recognition and appreciation that go beyond just feeling good. These benefits begin with team building.

Organizations that have a culture of recognition— especially peer-to-peer recognition—have strong bonds among team members. These organizations also have fewer problems with absenteeism. And they have stronger morale and better performance than organizations that don't have the same focus on recognition. When we feel like we're playing a vital and valued role we're more invested in our performance: We work harder, and we're likely to stick around longer.

Humor lets us build rapport with everyone we work with. And believe me, a wise nurse knows you never want to make an enemy of a CNA or someone from housekeeping . . . These unsung heroes play a pivotal role in making sure everything runs smoothly.

> *Humor helps some people reduce their bad cholesterol (LDL) while increasing their good cholesterol (HDL).*

Recognition has some serious benefits, but that doesn't mean you can't have fun with the process. In fact, light-hearted and humorous forms of appreciation are often the most well received. And they are easy to incorporate into even the busiest of environments.

Appreciation tends to work best when it's personally relevant.

One unit has a silver tiara (from Disneyland) at the nurses station. When one of the nurses solves a difficult problem or overcomes a real challenge, she is bestowed the tiara, and is crowned "Queen for the Day." (There's a "crab-hat" at the nurses station, too . . . But that's *another* story!)

One ambulatory clinic in San Diego has a "Surf Monkey"—dressed in scrubs, of course—that is passed from team member to team member every month, and each person is recognized for what he or she does. Posing with the Surf Monkey and having their picture posted prominently in the break room is part of the tradition. [Don't know what a Surf Monkey is? Go to Google Images for a chuckle!]

Look for opportunities to create your own organization-specific recognition traditions. One outpatient surgery team in Florida has a bright pink plastic lawn flamingo—dressed in surgical scrubs, of course—that they pass among team members monthly. Posing with the flamingo for photos is considered a great honor.

6. Create Shared History with Humor

"Otis elevator," said the surgeon. Nothing. The surgeon raised his eyebrow at the fledgling circulating nurse. "We need an *Otis elevator* in here!"

Bob, the circulating nurse, peered frantically at the instrument tray. Nothing. Panicked—but trying desperately not to show it—he headed out of the OR suite to locate the elusive 'Otis' elevator. He'd almost made it out the door before a kind-hearted nurse stopped him and explained, "It's a joke. He's teasing you!

'Otis' is the name of the company that makes the elevators that you ride up-and-down in—get it?"

This type of gentle teasing often serves as a rite of passage for new members of a healthcare team. The close bonds and tight relationships so characteristic of an OR team don't happen overnight. They take nurturing and cultivation. Sending a new team member to the lab for a "blue fallopian tube"—where the lab folks, understanding what's going on, will invariably reply that they only have *red* fallopian tubes—is a welcoming process. The use of humor is one way groups signal to new members that they are accepted, that they belong.

Here's a great rite of passage story from the world of long-term care:

It was the end of my first week of orientation, and I was beginning to think I had a good handle on my new job. The residents were all nice enough. A few had their issues, of course, but overall they were a good bunch. One thing that they all had in common, and what really got to me at first, was how hungry these folks were for attention and companionship.

They really wanted visits from their family, from their friends... It broke my heart to see how much.

One resident in particular, Irene, really got to me. I was getting ready to leave for the day when she said, "Can you do me a favor, honey? Can you sing me *Happy Birthday*? Tomorrow's my birthday and I don't think anyone is going to remember."

So I sang *Happy Birthday* to her. After a little conversation I found out that Irene really liked chocolate cake with butter cream frosting. So even though the next day was my day off, I baked a chocolate cake with butter cream frosting. Then I bought some balloons, and I delivered them to Irene. My colleagues smiled. Some of them nodded knowingly. I was happy that I was fitting-in so well.

On Monday my supervisor took me aside and said, "You made a lovely gesture on Saturday. But you need to know it wasn't Irene's birthday. Her birthday is actually four months away." I was confused.

She continued: "But Irene *loves* chocolate cake with butter cream frosting. And so, every time we get a new nurse, she pulls this little stunt on them."

My face burned red with embarrassment. I smacked my hand against my forehead and let out a groan. "Ugh. How many of them fall for it?" I asked.

"All the good ones," my supervisior smiled. "All the good ones."

If only all of the lessons that experience teaches us were this tasty! I love this story for so many reasons. First and foremost it reminds us that we must never forget that our patients are people first. There's nowhere on the chart to record the fact that Irene has a passionate sweet tooth, and flexible ethics when cake is on the line . . . But the nurse telling the tale will never forget.

Second, this story is a good illustration of one of the most common nursing experiences—the trial by fire. There are so many 'firsts' in nursing: Your first truly difficult patient, your first administrative snafu of epic proportions, your first time clearing out a crowded restaurant with nursing shop talk. We all have our stories of the first time. Some of these stories are funny. Some are touching. Some are sad. It's the nature of nursing.

Being able to bond over the 'birthday' cake gave this LTC nurse a quick, easy, and safe way to connect with her colleagues over a common experience. And if Irene enjoyed the balloons and chocolate cake with butter cream frosting, so much the better!

7. Fight Back Against Bullies with Humor

The room was thick with tension. A doctor, frustrated with his patient's failure to respond to treatment, started venting his anger on the nearest nurse. Taken aback, she stood there and took it for a moment. But then the doc's attack became intense and inappropriately personal.

And that's when the nurse called a *Code White*.

You may not be familiar with a Code White, but every nurse in *this* hospital was. Every available nurse on the floor came running. Like a football huddle, they gathered around the doctor and the nurse. And they simply stood there, silently bearing witness to what was happening.

It took a moment, but then through the haze of fury that had clouded his senses, the doctor became aware of the sea of nurses around him. His rant trailed off into silence. He cleared his throat, apologized, and slowly walked off the unit.

The Code White strategy was one healthcare team's response to workplace bullying. This informal procedure was very effective, as it is rooted in shaming behaviors—one of the oldest, most proven forms of social control. Other workplaces have more formal responses to workplace bullying. It's important to know what resources are available to you.

We've all been inundated with messages about how harmful bullying can be. School children often get the

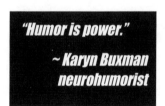

"Humor is power."

~ Karyn Buxman
neurohumorist

worst of it, but the abuse—which can be both physical and verbal—doesn't magically stop when kids turn 18. People who have learned that they can get their way by acting badly often continue acting badly until they encounter a compelling reason to change their behavior.

Some bullies grow up to be doctors. Some bullies grow up to be managers. Some bullies grow up to be patients. Some bullies even grow up to be nurses.

Where does that leave us? It's important to remember that we always have a choice in how we respond to a situation. The first experience with a bully may leave you feeling like you've been punched in the stomach, but you don't need to stay in that traumatized space.

It's also important to know how you can address your own personal reaction to being bullied. There's a five-step process that can help you transition from a state of shock to a state in which you can laugh and move past the bully's behavior.

Stage 1: Sad/Hurt/Shocked

Our initial reaction to being bullied is to feel hurt. Some people feel sad. And some are shocked. Many people just stand there and take it. Sometimes you simply don't know *how* to react. Especially if the bully is someone you respect and/or admire. And sometimes the power imbalance makes it nearly impossible to respond. (What if I look foolish? Will the abuse get worse? Could I lose my job?)

Stage 2: Anger & Hostile Humor

After we're done being shocked and hurt, we often move into being angry. And it's important to remember that being angry is a natural response. You're not a bad person or a bad nurse if you're angry after being bullied!

This is the stage where hostile humor comes easily. Think about jokes rooted in someone's ethnicity, appearance, or identity. When we're angry, we may use humor to vent—and it can be very easy for this humor to lead us to express ourselves in ways we otherwise would not.

Yes, anger has its place, but you don't want to *stay* angry. Anger is a burden, adding an additional layer of stress to your already busy day.

There is a Zen parable about . . .

> . . . Two monks—and old master, and a young novice—were traveling through the mountains. These monks were supposed to be chaste, having nothing at all to do with women.
>
> When the monks reached a wide river, they found a beautiful woman crying by the shore. She couldn't get across. The older monk picked her up, carried her across the river, set her down on the other side, and continued on his way.
>
> The younger monk followed him, but was greatly disturbed by what the older

> monk had done. He pondered it for a day and a night. He became increasingly upset . . . and he finally asked the older monk why he had helped the woman.
>
> The older monk smiled and said, "You are still carrying her? I left her back on the riverbank yesterday."

Anger is much the same. It can only affect us as long as we carry it with us. To move on, we have to be able to leave our fury behind us, on the river bank.

Stage 3: Pity/Contempt

As we contemplate the bully and what motivates him to act the way he does, we often find that it's obvious he's acting out of feelings of inferiority or insecurity. We may be moved to feel pity for these individuals. We also may feel contempt for them. Either way, we are moving away from a stage where we feel that the bully has the power to affect how we feel about ourselves. Instead, we're moving to a point where we see the sad source of bad behavior.

Stage 4: Indifference/Detachment

We feel nothing toward the bully. Her actions simply do no matter to us in the great scheme of things.

This type of detachment is difficult to reach the first time around: You may find yourself working through the five stages repeatedly before you can become indifferent to how someone conducts themselves.

Understand that achieving indifference is not the same thing as turning a blind eye to bad behavior. A person who is indifferent to a bully on a personal level may still be very motivated to have that bully's behavior addressed by the powers that be for reasons of team morale and improved patient care. We've all had the experience of having patients or their family members who forget to use their manners—yet we still provide consistently top-notch professional care.

If, as professionals, we can come from a place of empathy—stepping into the other person's shoes—we will be better able to recognize poor behavior as inappropriate, but not take it personally.

Stage 5: Positive Humor

When you've reached the point where the bully's behavior becomes a source of humor and amusement to you, you gain all of the healing benefits of laughter. This is the therapeutic stage, where humor helps you regain emotional balance and professional confidence. With practice, you'll find that turning to humor becomes easier and easier. This helps you preserve your emotional resources, so you can stay strong and focused in even the most challenging workplace environment.

My research proves that this works. And so does my professional life . . .

> As a young nurse, I was routinely bullied by a nurse manager. She made condescending remarks about me in front of the senior staff members on the floor.
>
> There were many days when I cried in the safety and privacy of my car, while driving home from work.
>
> And then . . . One day the light bulb came on. I realized what a miserable and insecure person the manager must be to pick on a newbie who felt powerless to protect herself.
>
> The next time she made a degrading comment, I visualized her as a little girl throwing a tantrum. Without even being aware of it at first, a smile of amusement came came over my face. I realized what

had happened when I saw the startled look on her face as she slowly backed away.

Changing my perspective, and finding the humor in the situation, had empowered me!

And here's the take-away: Bullies rarely pick on empowered people.

8. Keep Your Head When the S*** Hits the Fan

Through the course of your career as a nurse, things will happen which nothing—and I mean absolutely *nothing!*—you learned in nursing school has prepared you for . . .

[Another honest-to-goodness Real Life Story from the Files of Karyn Buxman, RN] . . .

To this day, I remember the shocked, stunned silence that filled the operating suite when the surgeon dropped the vein he'd just spent a whole hour harvesting from the patient's leg to use for a graft. The vein flipped out of his hand, did a 360 in the air, and then flopped onto the floor.

At a moment like this, nothing is funny. It's such a surreal moment. Had everyone not been wearing a mask, you would have seen a roomful of gaping mouths.

Once the vein had been retrieved, rinsed thoroughly and "blessed" with Betadine, and the procedure was completed successfully, the surgeon and the rest of the team needed to deal with the emotions that accompanied such an unexpected turn of events.

Once the shock wore off, we laughed at the sheer absurdity of the situation. In such a technologically and medically advanced setting, who would have thought that a simple case of butterfingers could cause so much drama?

And we laughed and laughed in sheer relief that everything turned out okay after all.

[If you haven't experienced this particular phenomenon for yourself, check out Season 1, Episode 1.9 of *Chicago Hope*, titled "Heartbreak."]

If you find yourself or your colleagues laughing in the aftermath of such an event, try to remember that this is a healthy way to process complex emotions.

Some people may be able to laugh immediately after something bad happens. For other people, it may take a little time.

And sometimes when the caca hits the fan, it's your quick thinking that will save the day. It may not be funny while you're living through it—but I guarantee that you'll laugh about it *later* . . .

> As a new grad, I felt excited and proud to assume the important responsibilities and tasks of an RN. One evening in our small hospital in Hannibal, Missouri, I learned what people mean when they say, "Sink or swim"!
>
> I was notified that a young man would be coming in for an emergency appendectomy, and I was to start his IV line. WOW! My first real IV without an instructor hovering over me.
>
> I carefully assembled my materials and then greeted my patient. He was a burly young man of about 25 with veins the size of garden hoses. The only drawback was his wife, who sat at the bedside,

scrutinizing my every move. Well, no problem, I was used to being observed.

I prepared my fluids and tubing, tore my tape, applied the tourniquet and prepared my IV site. I drew a deep breath, and then smoothly inserted the angiocath into the bulging vein. *Jackpot!* I connected the tubing, secured it, taped the site, and adjusted my flow rate. Feeling extremely successful (and just a tad smug), I turned to the wife and said, "Everything is going fine."

She crossed her arms and asked, "When are you going to take *that* off?" and pointed to the tourniquet.

I felt my stomach tightened and I broke out ito a cold sweat as I looked over to see the tourniquet *still wrapped tightly around my patient's now blue-tinged arm.*

My unconscious mind must have shifted into high gear. Without missing a beat I smiled . . . I held my watch up in front of me . . . I reached over with my other hand and grabbed the end of the

tourniquet . . . and, with my eyes fixed on
my watch, I calmly said, "I can take it off
. . . [pause] . . . right . . . [pause] . . . *now*."
I then snapped the tourniquet off with a
professional (if dramatic) flourish.

Whew! My humor and wit allowed me to maintain
my sense of control and save face in front of my
patient, while maintaining the patient's confidence in me!

9. Upping Others' Attitudes—By Upping Yours

"A loving person lives in a loving world. A hostile
person lives in a hostile world. Everyone you meet is
your mirror." [I wish I'd coined this thought. But alas,
it was Ken Keyes, and expert on happiness.] Our
experiences are affected by our attitudes and beliefs.

What does this mean? Obviously, we don't have
the ability to control how other people conduct themselves. [Life would be *so* much easier if people would
act the way *we* wanted them to! But alas.]

But while we can't *control* other people, we do have
the ability to *influence* how they act. The way we do that
is, as Keyes suggests, with our own behavior. It's an
easy theory to test:

On Day One, smile at everyone you see. Take note
of how many people smile back, or are cheerful and
happy in your presence.

And then, on Day Two, frown at everyone you see. Again, take note of how people react. You'll hear a lot more complaining and negativity when you greet the world with a negative expression. There's a lot of fascinating research being conducted regarding the complex social and physiological reasons why this phenomenon happens, but there's no arguing that it does happen.

Chances are that your day as a nurse would be far more pleasant and satisfying if you were surrounded by people who were, by and large, in a good mood and happy to see you. You can stack the deck in favor of this happening by being in a good mood yourself. Humor plays a huge role in this. Learning to see and appreciate the funny moments in life makes it easier to keep smiling. Sharing humor makes other people happier as well. And happier people are nicer to be around, and ergo, your day gets better.

[Ta-daa!]

"Humor is a rubber sword.

It allows you to make a point

without drawing blood."

~ MARY HIRSCH

Chapter 6
So . . . What IS so Funny About Nursing?

We've talked about the patient. We've talked about the team you work with. Now it's time to talk about *you*, the nurse.

Our profession has many rewards. It also has many challenges. In order to thrive, personally and professionally, it's essential that we take an active role in our own self-care. We can't count on others to provide the support and validation we need.

Self-care isn't always easy. Living a healthy and balanced life is an admirable goal—but it's not a goal that's necessarily compatible with being a nurse. Sure, a healthy diet is important—but after a week of 12-hour shifts who has the energy to go grocery shopping, much less cook?!

Anyway, the vending machines are filled with goodies from the four basic food groups: Caffeine, sugar, salt, and fat. One soon discovers that scrubs can effectively cover a multitude of sins—and pounds!

A Tweet regarding a nursing staff: "They're like seagulls. They'll eat anything."

Some nurses are fans of exercise as a stress-buster. I think every team has one of these folks—you know the type: She goes for a 12-mile run after a 12-hour shift. The rest of us mere mortals work up a sweat just *thinking* about it!

Some nurses are fans of chocolate and/or wine as stress-busters. Personally, I'm a fan of both. But, as in most things, moderation is wise.

And some of us are "fans of funny." Laughing is not only fun, but it's good for you! [This sounds like a TV jingle for some sugary cereal, doesn't it?!] Well, the fact is—and scientists have proven—that laughing has similar physiological benefits to plain old physical exercise. So if it's a choice between running a marathon, or participating in an *I Love Lucy* marathon—you'll find me on the couch, laughing [exercising!].

Laughter is easy. Laughter is fun. Laughter is energizing. Laughter is 100% portable. Laughter is available wherever you are. And . . . laughter is free! Cultivating the humor habit—learning to see the funny that surrounds us every day—makes every day as a nurse just a little bit easier. Laughter lifts the spirits, lowers stress levels, and restores emotional resiliency.

To be a happier, healthier, more effective nurse, laugh every day.

Following are many ways for you to make "finding the funny" a part of your daily routine. These techniques are simple, fast, cheap and fun.

Think of this as the Grand Buffet of

> *Laugher is good exercise. Really.*
>
> *Laughter is a universal lauguage—across cultures and across ages.*
>
> *Laughter is just plain fun!*

Humor. Take what you like and leave the rest! Don't feel obligated to pile everything onto your plate. [Good news: Unlike smorgasbords, excessive humor does not lead to "muffin tops."]

Humor is deeply personal. As you read through these pages, you'll find some techniques and strategies that make you laugh out loud, and you'll find others curious or just plain odd. You'll realize maximum benefits by choosing and practicing those techniques and strategies that resonate with you. If it makes you laugh, it's going to work.

Choose from among the following humor strategies the ones that you feel are fun and playful, that you simply enjoy, and that just make you laugh.

11 Humor Strategies to Help Nurses Keep their Sanity

1. Be a Humor Collector

The goal here is to laugh every day. The challenge is to figure out exactly how to make this happen. One thing I've found, over the course of more than two decades of focused research, is that the world is a really, really funny place. The trick is to keep your eyes open, pay attention, and be aware of the humorous things that are happening all around you.

Geneticists may not have found the "Collecting Gene" yet, but there's no arguing that for some people, searching for and finding the object of their desire is a large part of the fun. Fossil hunters spend hours happily hiking trails and riverbeds searching for their treasures. Art collectors are always on the hunt, going to galleries, shows, and studios in search of the Next

Big Thing. These activities add joy to their lives. Humor collecting works the same way—except you don't need to spend any money, and there's no hiking required!

I love how easy it is to build a Humor Collection using smart phones and computers. There are joke-of-the-day apps, funny blogs, and as many humorous books as you can load onto your Kindle. Create your own YouTube channel of funny videos. Set-up your Netflix queue with the best comedies ever.

And if you want to go Old School, save cartoons and jokes from the newspaper. Build a library of books by funny authors, collect comedy records. [Records?!! CDs? DVD's? MP3s? Holographic memories downloadable directly into your brain?]

Give yourself the freedom to create a humor collection that is wholly and completely your own. It's all about you! What makes you laugh? Remember, this is your own private source of amusement—if you're tickled beyond all reason by pictures of French Poodles driving cars, no one needs to know. [Your secret is safe with me!]

Finding items to put in your humor collection is only half the fun. The other half is experiencing these funny items again and again. Whenever you're feeling down, or in need of a smile, check out your humor collection. Something in there is sure to make you laugh. It's a fast way to lift your spirits.

Here's a piece to get you started:

You Know You're a Nurse When . . .

- You no longer giggle when a patient with multiple piercings and full-sleeve tattoos tells you she's afraid of needles.

- You fill-out 'frequent flier' medical histories from memory.

- When a patient tell you how many drinks he's had, you automatically triple the number.

- You make a point of making sure to use the bathroom every single day—whether you (with your Winnebago-sized bladder!) need to or not!

- You jingle when you walk . . . from all the scissors, keys and clamps in your pockets.

- You know that not all patients are annoying. Some are unconscious.

- You have the phone numbers of every late-night food delivery place in town memorized . . . But can't remember where you left your car keys.

- You can diagnosis illnesses solely by the smell of the diarrhea.

- You never, ever, *ever* answer your phone on your day off.

- It's been a year since you've seen a pen not imprinted with the name of a laxative or anti-depressant.

- Your finger has gone into places you never thought possible.

- You've ever wrapped a gift in a hospital pillowcase, secured with Micropore tape.

- Your sense of humor gets more warped every year.

2. Stay in the Moment

You can't text empathy and compassion to a patient.

Hey, I love my iPhone, too! It allows me to stay in close touch with clients, friends and family. I text, I tweet, I email, and heck, I even make phone calls!

And yet nothing takes the place of face-to-face interaction. With friends, and family, and especially with patients. There's a reason why nursing is called a "hands-on" profession. One of the things that distinguishes nursing from other branches of the healthcare world is that we maintin the high-touch in an increasingly high-tech profession.

Staying face-to-face with patients, and staying in the moment with them, is healing. And . . . humor works best when it is experienced first-hand, too.

3. Raise Your Awareness

Every day contains humor. It's just that on some days this humor is more apparent than on others. Sometimes laughter is easy to find. Sometimes you have to look for it. I refer to the strategy of actively seeking out humor as "Raising Awareness." Raising Awareness means choosing to recognize the funny side of life and deliberately cultivating laughter and mirth.

Practice asking yourself: "What is there to laugh about?" When you can do that on a daily basis, you will then have a skill that you can carry with you anywhere, and use any time. Using this skill will improve the quality of your work and your life.

Here's a secret that every comedian knows: It's a lot easier to *see* funny than to *be* funny. Seeing funny is one of the easiest ways to integrate humor into your life. In fact, once you start, you might not be able to stop!

"If I hadn't believed it, I wouldn't have seen it."

~ ASHLEIGH BRILLIANT

The first step in seeing funny is to believe that there is funny to be seen. If your worldview tells you that there's nothing funny happening in your life, then you'll be right. On the other hand, if you believe that the world is an amusing place just waiting for you to discover it, then you'll be right, too.

> It's not unusual for many of our patients to mispronounce the procedure they're having, or even the condition they have.
>
> Instead of a colonoscopy, one patient said that she was coming in for a "colostomy." Another woman thought that her surgery was for "very close veins." One athlete came into have his 'rotary cuff' fixed. One 81-year-old patient wondered why everyone on staff chuckled when she called her thoracentesis an "amniocentesis."
>
> But my absolute favorite is the little old lady who told me, with great enthusiasm, as we were walking her out from her breast biopsy, "Honey, that was the best autopsy I've ever had!"

[Thanks to Veronica Thomas, RN!]

And sometimes Raising Awareness merely means being open to recognizing humor when it presents itself—even if you can't laugh right that moment . . .

> I had a situation with a nursing student that was humorous after-the-fact. She was from a different culture than our patient population, and very stoic by nature.
>
> We had just covered Therapeutic Communication in class, and the student nurse proceeded to her first clinical day. She was caring for a very old woman with dementia. The woman had a moment of clarity and asked the student if she was going to die.
>
> The student matter-of-factly said, "Yes, you will. In fact, we all will." The patient burst into tears . . . And the student couldn't understand why. We had to revisit Therapeutic Communication strategies several more times before this student graduated!"

[Thanks to Beth Cusatis Phillips, MSN, RN, CNE!]

Let yourself believe that the world is full of humor. Just taking this simple step will place you light years ahead of those around you who are in too much of a hurry to take a moment to see and hear and experience the vast absurdity and delight going on all around us.

As one of the world's great philosophers once said:

"From there to here,
and here to there,
funny things are everywhere."

~ Dr. Seuss

How often have you heard something hysterical at work, but just couldn't remember it the next day? Well, one person who takes the time to record funny comments in the OR is @ORDailyQuote (a prolific tweeter). He's not necessarily a *creator* of humor, but he is an *observer* and *collector* of humor. ("I don't tell 'em what to say. I just quote 'em.") Further, he loves to share his humorous observations with the world.

Now, a lot of laymen won't get—or appreciate—

these observations, because there's a lot of insider humor here. But what the heck, it's all about *us*, isn't it?!

To wit:

- Surgeon: "Everyone say a prayer to the gods of homeostasis."
- ENT surgeon while making his incision: "A scar is born."
- Urologist: "It all comes down to the jerk at the end of the suture."
- Tech palpating a clotted AV fistula: "The thrill is gone."
- "I have angered the call gods, and I don't know how to appease them."
- Anesthesiologist, while performing a fiberoptic intubation and looking into the scope: "I think I see the Chilean miners!"
- RN: "He's throwing things at me!" Scrub tech: "No he's not. He's got better aim than that."
- Anesthesiologist: "Hope is not a plan."
- Scrub tech: "My pee smells like coffee."
- Circulating Nurse, regarding Scrub Nurse: "We call her by her Indian name, Running Commentary."

You, too, can follow our fellow recorder-of-OR-humor on Twitter at www.Twitter.com/ORDailyQuote.

And here are a few *more* tweets for your amusement:

- Overheard in the ER: "I drive way too fast to worry about cholesterol."
- You know you're a nurse when . . . Your family won't allow you to discuss your day at work at the dinner table . . . EVER!
- Facing your fears is great. But running from them makes for a great cardio workout.

Follow @FunnyNurse on Twitter for more insider humor, courtesy of JournalOfNursingJocularity.com.

4. Look for the Funny Around You: Visual Humor

Cartoons, comics and other funny pictures can provide almost instant laughs, and they're yours for the clipping. But don't stop there! To get more mileage out of the cartoons, personalize them! Write-in people's names or places of interest (surgeons, nurses, administrators—anyone's fair game, but it's a good idea to stick to people who have a good sense of humor). Tack the cartoons to the break room bulletin board.

Massage your creativity! White-Out the captions and let everyone come up with their own.

And to further stretch your brain: *The New Yorker*

magazine is well known for its cartoon caption contest, wherein the editors present readers with a cartoon without a caption. The challenge is to write your own caption, then submit it for possible publication. From thousands of submissions weekly, the editors choose their three favorites, then print them in the magazine; the public then votes for their favorites, and the winner becomes world-famous by having his or her caption featured in *The New Yorker!* (This could be something you do on your own—or something you brainstorm with your team.)

> **Humor boosts morale.**
>
> **Humor makes people more pleasant.**
>
> **Humor helps when things go wrong.**

[Don't get *The New Yorker?* Well, you can participate online. Visit www.NewYorker.com/humor/caption.]

Some great sources for nursing cartoons include JournalOfNursingJocularity.com (featuring the infamous "Nurse Marge in Charge"); Nurstoon.com (tons of nursing topics) by funnyman Carl Elbing; and ScrubsMagazine.com (featuring a variety of different cartoonists). You can also view tons of syndicated cartoons (Peanuts, Cathy, Blondie, Garfield, Ziggy, etc.) at GoComics.com. Or, if you just like dark humor in general, check out CallahanOnline.com!

5. LISTEN for the Funny Around You: Verbal Humor

Sharing verbal humor can be done in two ways. The first is telling jokes. The second is by sharing funny stories.

Jokes

If you hear a great joke, pass it on! Humor shared is humor increased.

Q: What's the difference between a surgeon and a puppy?
A: Eventually the puppy grows up and quits whining.

A word to the wise: When you don't know your audience well, stay away from political jokes, religious jokes, alcohol-related stories, racial observations, gender put-downs, yo-mama jokes, jokes in "bad taste" (although this is often hard to judge), and what most people would consider "sick humor."

Here are some stories and jokes that have been thoroughly tested and nurse-approved . . .

———————

A hospital posted a notice in the nurses' lounge that said: "Remember, the first five minutes of a human being's life are the most dangerous." Underneath, a nurse had written: "The last five are pretty risky, too."

Q: How do you scare a gynecologist?
A: Become a ventriloquist.

Q: Why do doctors dress so poorly?
A: Because pharmaceutical reps don't give away clothing.

There was a urologist who had a personalized license plate that read: 2PCME

Four doctors were out duck hunting on a lake. But it was open season for only one species of duck.

After many hours on the boat without seeing a single duck, they all dozed off.

The general practitioner awoke to see a whole flock of ducks flying overhead.

Unsure if they were the ducks currently in season, he roused and consulted with the specialist.

The specialist wasn't sure, so he woke up the surgeon. As soon as the surgeon saw the ducks, he started blasting away.

"Are you sure those ducks are in season?" the first two doctors asked.

The surgeon replied, "Wake the pathologist and ask *him!*"

Stories

Funny stories, drawn from our own experiences, can help us build strong bonds with the people we work with. More than that, they're fun to tell. Your colleagues will laugh, and you get to laugh along with them, experiencing all of the mental and physical benefits of humor.

Laughing provides a sense of control.

Humor helps people perservere.

Humor provides a safe space to process emotions.

If you want to really connect with people, you may want to develop your skills at story telling. As they say, practice makes perfect. (Note: It is easier to tell a *story* well than it is to tell a *joke* well.)

Become a collector of stories. Seek them from the people you work with every day. Ask what their favorite funny memory is, what makes them laugh, what's their most embarrassing moment.

You'll get two benefits from doing this. First, others will see you as a humorous person. And second, you'll now have a repertoire of stories that you can share with others.

Here's a funny story told to me by a nurse at a healthcare conference:

> During a recent fire drill, I was closing doors to patients' rooms. An 86-year-old patient was talking on the phone when I reached her room.
>
> As I started to close her door, she asked me, "What's that ringing noise?"
>
> "Don't worry," I answered, "We're just having a little fire drill."
>
> The patient turned back to her call. As I was leaving I heard her say, "No, everything's just fine, dear. The hospital's on fire but a nice nurse just came to lock me in my room."

There are some stories that are universal. People are people no matter where you go, and they keep finding the same ways to trip and slip, twist and shout, crash and burn.

Every team—every doctor, nurse and tech, in fact—will have their own versions of these stories. One classic tale is the "You have *what* lodged *where*??" story. [I'm not judging—just observing.] In fact, there's an entire book devoted to this topic: *Stuck Up! 100 Objects Inserted and Ingested Where They Shouldn't Be.* [You *really* don't have to make this stuff up . . .]

> **Laughter lightens one's mood.**
>
> **Humor supports intimacy.**
>
> **Frivolity reduces fear.**

Another story shared by many nurses is the "Funniest thing I ever heard a patient say" or "Funniest thing I ever saw a patient do" tale. These stories aren't intended to poke fun at our patients but to acknowledge the many ridiculous, absurd moments that happen in healthcare like:

- Encountering a patient who is wandering around, completely naked.
- Listening to a patient complaining that his pill tasted awful—only to discover that it was a suppository.
- Discovering your NPO patient had a pizza delivered to his room.

6. Play Around!

Playful people are happier people. Happy people are healthier people. This is true for everyone, but it's especially true for nurses. One of the best ways to introduce humor into your day, and become a happier, stronger, calmer caregiver is to embrace the power of play.

Playing, having fun, using your imagination . . . once upon a time, these were our only jobs in the world. When we were kids, life was all about playing. Then, as adult responsibilities began piling up, less and less time became available for playing. We've gotten too busy to have fun.

"We do not stop playing because we grow old; we grow old because we have stopped playing."

~ Benjamin Franklin

The time for play may have disappeared, but the need for it has not. We need our imagination, our silliness, our make-believe and clever games, just as much as we did when we were kids. Perhaps even more. Play is incredibly powerful—it lifts the spirit, rejuvenates and energizes, and adds a much-needed element of joy to our days.

Play is very important, and yet it is almost universally undervalued. Trust me, I've been paying attention . . . to children, to adults, to patients with many conditions, and to the medical and scientific journals.

Because children play, we consider play to be a childish thing. Yet nothing could be further from the truth. Play can transform the way we see the world. And let's be real here—after a long day at

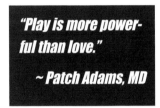

"Play is more powerful than love."

~ Patch Adams, MD

work, sometimes our worldview could use a little transformation!

Here's one way you can incorporate the power of play into your life: Create a "Play List," full of things that are fun for you to do! It can include playing games, playing sports, playing piano, playing with your kids, playing with your dog (or your kids' dogs, or your dog's kids). At least half your list should be low-cost or no-cost [unless you're both rich *and* a nurse, in which case, go wild!].

When you're feeling down, or it's been a really bad day, do at least one thing on your Play List. There is a method to the madness here. Those times when you are most in need of play, are the times when you are least able to think of something fun to do. When you're feeling sick or tired or frustrated, nothing sounds like much fun.

So don't wait until you feel better to do the things on your Play List! That would be missing the point. Let play transform your crummy day. Perform an activity from your Play List when you're feeling bad, and I promise you'll feel better.

"What if the Hokey-Pokey really *is* what it's all about?"
~ Bumper sticker

[Because really . . . Is it possible to have a bad day while doing the Hokey-Pokey??]

Bingo!

Put the power of play to work by bringing your whole team on board. Even the simplest game can get your team laughing, boosting the group's morale.

One great way to involve the team in play is a little game I created: "What's So Funny About... Nursing BINGO!"

What's so Funny About... Nursing? Bingo

Can't Find My Pen	NPO Patient Eats	Simultaneous Codes	Empty Linen Cart	I&O Pt Empties Own Urinal
Change of Shift Admission	Projectile Vomit	Patient Left AMA	IV Won't Stop Beeping	Can't Find Patient
Family Gifts Nurses: Chocolate	Patient Has 6+ Visitors	Free Bingo Space!	Code Brown	Naked Patient in Hall
Family Member c/o Doctor	Coffee Pot Is Empty	2 Nurses Call in Sick	Working Overtime	Doctor Says Thank You!
Catch Pt Smoking in BR	Can't Find a Wheelchair	Mandatory Inservice	Student Nurse Assigned	No Time to Pee

Scan this code with your smartphone to find a downloadable version of this bingo card and learn other ways to improve global health through humor and laughter.

Scan the QR code or go to . . .

http://karynbuxman.com/wp-content/uploads/ WSFA_Nursing_BingoWhite.pdf . . . to print copies for your whole team. Play traditional, or four corners, or blackout—your choice. And, of course, there must be prizes of unspeakable value for the winners (things like gummy bears, costume jewelry, marbles, Legos, balloons, bagels, funny buttons, loose change or lottery tickets).

7. Laugh for No Reason Whatsoever, a.k.a. Laughter Yoga

What kind of health book would this be if it didn't include at least a passing nod to exercise?! Any time I want to get a group of nurses laughing, I recommend a vigorous workout routine of early morning runs, followed by mid-afternoon aerobics, and evening spin classes. This schedule alone is enough to reduce some of you to tears (of laughter).

That's great news, because experts have discovered that even fake laughter has benefits! [No, really!]

Charles Schaefer, a psychology professor at Fairleigh Dickinson University, conducted a study demonstrating that even completely fake laughter can boost mood and overall well-being. In the study, participants were asked to laugh heartily for one full minute. Afterward, they reported feeling better, and having a more positive outlook on life. The study was repeated with similar results, and has inspired the creation of many laughter groups.

Laughter clubs can be found in many locations across the country and aroud the world. These can be a great resource, offering a chance to connect with other like-minded individuals. You can learn more by visiting WorldLaughterTour.com to find existing groups or to learn how to form your own laughter club.

Here are some laughter exercises you can try (and these will all work in the privacy of your own home, in case you're uncomfortable looking silly in public).

Ice Cube Laughter

Pretend that someone has dropped an ice cube down the back of your shirt. How would your body react? Hop up-and-down, reach behind you to try and remove the ice cube. Shake, jump, shiver and wiggle while you giggle!

Electric Shock Laughter

Pretend you're getting an electric shock from everything you touch. Give a great big exaggerated response to every pretend shock: Jump up in the air, wave your arms, yell "Ay Caramba!" It won't take long before you're laughing like crazy!

Hula Hoop Laughter

Imagine a Hula Hoop around your hips. Get the hoop moving by swinging your hips in a circular motion, and laugh while you keep the hoop moving.

Hearty Laughter

Laugh while raising both arms toward the sky with your head tilted a little bit backwards. Feel as if the laughter is coming from your heart. Laugh as loud as you can, for as long as you can. It may feel forced at first, but soon you'll find yourself genuinely laughing.

Gradient Laughter

Start by smiling—then slowly begin to laugh with a gentle chuckle. Increase the intensity and volume of the laugh until you've achieved a robust laugh. Then gradually bring the laugh back down to a smile again.

8. Take the 24-Hour Challenge

If you want to increase the amount of laughter in your life, not to mention the physical and mental benefits associated with humor, I invite you to try the 24-Hour Challenge.

It's really simple. When you find something that makes you laugh out loud, you have 24 hours to share that experience with someone else. Sometimes this is easy. See a split-your-sides picture on Facebook? Share it with your friends. If it makes you laugh, chances are it will make other people laugh as well.

Hear a great joke? Tell it to the next person you meet. See a really funny film? Take your spouse or partner to see it, too. When we laugh with someone, we become closer to that person. Humor creates bonds and connections between us. It's a positive experience that rejuvenates and refreshes.

One of the great side benefits of sharing humor with others is that they're encouraged to share humor with you. When people know that you appreciate a good joke, they'll make a point of telling you good jokes they've heard. You've established yourself as a receptive audience for humor—and you get to reap the rewards in laughter.

Another way to approach the 24-Hour Challenge is to commit to making one person laugh every single day. It's a simple little habit, but one that can have a tremendous impact on your quality of life—and theirs!

Let's face it. There are some days when being a nurse is not only hard, it's demoralizing. Things—heartbreaking things—can happen, and there's nothing you can do about them. So many things are out of our control. But we *can* control is how we interact with the people around us. When we make someone else smile, it's going to make us smile—and that tiny little boost to our spirit and psyche can give us the critical resiliency we need to come back and do the same thing all over again tomorrow.

So don't forget: Humor shared is humor increased. [It's too bad chocolate doesn't work like that!]

9. Decorate for Laughs

Everyone is intensely affected by the environment in which they live. Let's define "living space" as any location where you spend large amounts of time, which includes both home and work. Your living space has a huge impact on the way you view the world and yourself.

Elements of the healthcare setting are by design cold, clean, and sterile. It's an environment created to facilitate focus and control. There's no place for distraction; things are kept simple and clean for infection control. And many times, we're working in an environment relatively low on visual stimuli, with a relatively bland color scheme of chrome, white or seafoam-green, and tile.

There's not much that can be done about this. However, it's important to recognize and honor the role our environment has on our psyche. There's no law that says you can't decorate areas such as the break room to lighten your mood. It doesn't take much. Some funny cartoons can be enough to bring a smile to your face. Or, if your team has a "mascot," you might want to keep it where everyone can see it. I've seen lawn flamingos, stuffed polar bears, and even a Tickle-Me-Elmo serving as team mascots.

Another fun idea is to collect pictures of the team and their pets. Post them separately and see if you can match-up the pairs that belong together. [Some people really *do* look like their dogs. Be prepared. You'll never look at a Chihuahua or Shih Tzu the same way again!]

You can even decorate *yourself.* When taking care of patients in isolation, I was known to take a magic marker to decorate my mask with a smile, or to draw bling on my disposable gloves. My lab coat generally sported buttons with humorous messages, like "Stop me before I become my mother!" or "What's wrong? Is it my hair?" or "You have something stuck between your teeth."

One facility even held a hospital-wide contest for their employees: Bedpan Hat Decorations! The hospital provided participants with clean, never-before-used bedpans. The participants provided the creativity, crayons, flowers, streamers, buttons, Slinkeys, tubing, etc.

10. Let the Music Move You

Music is a powerful tool that can lift your mood, elevate your spirits, and positively impact your emotional state. Nurses, anesthetists, and doctors have combined their healthcare expertise with their musical talents to create some unique entertainment.

You may want to try introducing some of these tunes by creating a fun playlist.

Too Live Nurse (a.k.a., the RNs of Rock) provides stress relief and entertainment with songs and parodies such as "The Girl with Emphysema," "Doin' The Incontinence Rag," and "Ventilate Me."

Deb Gauldin, "The Singing Nurse," inspires and entertains fellow nurses with songs like, "I Wanted to be Florence Nightingale," "PMS Blues," and "With a Little Help from Depends."

Another ensemble, Dr. Sam and The Managed Care Blues Band, sings about serious healthcare issues with witty tunes like "Capitation Blues," "Managed Healthcare Blues," and "You Picked a Fine Time to Leave Me, Blue Shield."

And, of course, there's the Laryngospasms, a group of nurse anesthetists, who combine their sense of humor and musical talents to bring you medical parodies of classic and familiar songs such as "Anesthesia Dreamin'," "Waking Up Is Hard to Do," and "The Little Old Lady with Her Fractured Femur."

11. Find Someone Who "Gets It"

One of the hazards of being a nurse is that you're privy to all kinds of hysterically funny things that happen in the course of a day—and there are very few people in the world who will find those things funny, too. Sure, spouses and partners try, and your friends will indulge you every now and then—but frankly, a lot of what's funny about nursing has to do with blood, boogers, and body fluids. This isn't material that everyone is comfortable thinking about, much less laughing about. Another nurse, however, will know where you're coming from.

ENT surgeon (during sinus surgery): "That's a lotta boogers."
OR nurse: "No it's snot."

Humor researchers talk about the phenomenon of "insider humor." This is humor that comes from shared experiences. If you haven't had the experience, you might "understand" the joke—but you probably won't find it funny. In fact, you may judge it to be inappropriate, gross or just plain mean.

That's why one healthcare team I know created a "Dilly Code." This is a private [shhh!] code, the significance of which is known only to team personnel. When a Dilly Code is called, all available team members converge on a secret location, snack on Dilly Bars (a Dairy Queen specialty), and [are you ready?? . . .] just shoot the breeze. (The result? Stress reduction. Stronger bonds. More community. And laughs. Lots and lots of laughs.) Ten minutes spent laughing with your colleagues can have a significant positive impact on everyone's day.

Another way to find professional "soul mates" (those who "get it") is to form friendships with other nurses, locally and nationally. Professional association meetings and conventions offer prime opportunities to meet people who have the same sense of humor that you do. Make a point of connecting online, on the phone, or in person, at least every few weeks.

Social media can also provide some great opportunities for sharing your sense of humor when your family thinks you're crazy. One nurse-oriented Facebook source is FB.com/JournalOfNursing Jocularity. And some Twitter sources include @ORDailyQuotes and @FunnyNurse. (Additional resources are listed at the back of this book.)

Five minutes spent laughing with someone who understands can do more than just lift your mood. It's a solid reminder that you're not alone. Other nurses are facing the same challenges and obstacles that you are. Working together—and laughing together—makes it easier for all of us.

"Life should be lived as play."

~ PLATO

Chapter 7
The Last Laugh

As a nurse, humorist and professional speaker who spends a lot of time traveling, I have to say I love Southwest Airlines. These folks use applied humor to keep a group of people who are in a relatively high-stress situation moving, on-task, and generally pleasant. When the flight attendant starts the safety check with the line, "There may be 50 ways to leave your lover, but there's only four ways to leave this plane . . ." people laugh—but they also pay attention.

There's another line I heard from a Southwest flight attendant, and it's particularly important information if you happen to be a nurse. The flight attendant had reached the part of the safety instructions where she was detailing what would happen in the unlikely event that the plane loses cabin pressure. Oxygen masks would drop down from the ceiling. We could don them, she explained, if continuing to breathe fit into our plans for the afternoon.

That's when she said the magic line. "If you're traveling with a child, or someone behaving like a child, *make sure to put your own oxygen mask on first!*"

Ladies and gentlemen, truer words were never spoken. Put your own oxygen mask on first. You have to take care of yourself before you can take care of other people.

> *"Nurses must take care of ourselves first before we can take care of others."*
>
> ~ KAREN DALEY, PhD, MPH, RN, FAAN
> PRESIDENT OF THE AMERICAN NURSES ASSOCIATION

Before we do what we do to change our patients' lives for the better, we need to make sure we're looking out for our own physical and emotional health, too. No one is going to do this for us. We need to do it for ourselves.

One great way to do this is to start every day with a laugh—or two. Make humor as important to your morning routine as that first cup of coffee. Before heading out the door, check-out the silly pictures your friends have posted on Facebook. Goof around with your kids before they leave for school. Find a funny drive-time radio show to enjoy. These daily morning laughs make up your own personal oxygen mask. Make sure you put it on!

And so . . . To send you on your way with a smile on your face—here's my all-time-favorite nurse joke:

Three doctors are walking on a beach. They spot a magic lamp and one of them picks it up and rubs it. Out pops a genie who says, "I'll grant each of you one wish!"

The pediatrician smiles and says, "Make me 25% smarter then these guys."

The genie looks at him, nods, and says, "Your wish is granted! You are now *25% smarter.*"

The cardiologist chuckles and says, "Make me 50% smarter than these guys."

The genie looks at him, nods, and says, "Your wish is granted! You are now *50% smarter.*"

The neurosurgeon smirks and says, "Make me *100%* smarter than these guys."

The genie looks at him, nods, and says, "Your wish is granted! You are now . . . *a nurse!*"

4 out of 5 doctors recommend

Online resources can deepen your understanding of applied and therapeutic humor for nurses.

Association for Applied & Therapeutic Humor, www.aath.org

This non-profit organization serves as the community for professionals who study, practice and promote healthy humor. (Non-professionals love it, too.) Includes a monthly ezine, teleconferences, annual conference, CEs, and graduate credit via the Humor Academy.

Comic-Con, www.Comic-Con.org

An annual gathering of 140,000 fans of popular culture, including movie fans, sci-fi fans, Star Wars aficionados, super hero lovers, and comic book fans.

FunnyNurse, www.Twitter.com/FunnyNurse

Humor for nurses in 140 characters or less. Caution: May contain references to body fluids, death, & dismemberment.

GoComics, www.GoComics.com

Lots and lots (and lots) of your favorite syndicated comic strips. [Peanuts and Cathy and Ziggy, oh my!]

Journal of Nursing Jocularity
www.JournalOfNursingJocularity.com
Humor by nurses for nurses. An online salute to the magazine published from 1991-1998 by Doug Fletcher, RN.

www.Facebook.com/JournalOfNursingJocularity
A Facebook group where nurses can share their humorous experiences and observations.

Laughter Yoga www.LaughterYoga.org
Founded by Dr. Madan Kataria, Laughter Yoga combines unconditional laughter with yogic breathing (Pranayama). Exercises, events, and information.

The New Yorker Cartoon Caption Contest
www.newyorker.com/humor/caption
A weekly contest where anyone can submit captions to a cartoon provided by *The New Yorker*. The winners' captions appear in the magazine. No cash prizes, but it's great for bragging rights!

O.R. Quotes, www.Twitter.com/ORDailyQuote
Real quotes from a real operating room.

Songs for Unsung Heroes,
www.DebGauldin.com/products
Humorous and inspiring songs *for* nurses, *by* a nurse.

Pintereset Nurse Humor
www.Pinterest.com/KarynBuxman/nurse-humor
Funny images and videos that you can re-pin to create your own nurse humor collection.

StoryPeople, www.StoryPeople.com
Unique and playful illustrations, artwork, physical and electronic greeting cards with funny and/or insightful thoughts, by artist/poet Brian Andreas.

What's So Funny About$^{®}$ . . .?
www.WhatsSoFunnyAbout.com
Ongoing information on applied and therapeutic humor for chronic illnesses, including heart disease, diabetes, cancer, Alzheimer's, depression, and more— by Karyn Buxman, RN.

World Laughter Tour
www.WorldLaughterTour.com
Founded by Steve Wilson and Karyn Buxman to support, promote, and act as a clearinghouse for the global laughter movement, with the mission of bringing events to every continent that supports health and peace through laughter. Articles, exercises, news and events.

Books by Karyn Buxman

What's So Funny About . . . Diabetes?

What's So Funny About . . . Heart Disease?

What's So Funny About . . . OR Nursing?

What's So Funny About . . . School Nursing?

Amazed & Amused

Laughing Your Way to More Money, Better Sex & Thinner Thighs

Humor Me (co-author)

The Service Prescription (co-author)

Chicken Soup for the Nurses Soul (contributor)

Coming soon in the "What's So Funny About...?" series

What's So Funny About . . . Alzheimer's?

What's So Funny About . . . Cancer?

What's So Funny About . . . Depression?

What's So Funny About . . . Parkinson's?

What's So Funny About . . . Aging?

What's So Funny About . . . Dialysis?

What's So Funny About . . . Love?

Karyn Buxman, RN, MSN, CSP, CPAE

The Really Important Stuff

Karyn Buxman is an RN with attitude . . . and a serious sense of humor. As a nurse, she cared for hundreds of patients one-on-one; as a motivational keynoter, she now administers to thousands of people from the stage. Karyn is a neurohumorist—one who researches the neurobiology of humor, and then translates these cutting-edge findings for the layperson, showing how they can harness applied humor to heal and empower themselves.

Karyn presents laughter with a purpose. Mirth with a message. Humor that heals. Keynotes that enlighten, educate and entertain. Karyn's key messages are: "Humor is power" — "You don't need to BE funny—just SEE funny" — "Humor by CHANCE is *funny*. But humor by CHOICE is *life-changing*." Karyn has been described as "One part Norman Cousins, one part Patch Adams, and two parts Lucille Ball."

The Additional Stuff

But wait—there's more! . . . There's that mind-body-spirit connection thing! As a researcher *and* performer, Karyn brings science, psychology and humor to health, success and spirituality.

What else? . . . Karyn has addressed 5,000 members of the Million Dollar Roundtable in Thailand; rocked 8,500 OR nurses in Chicago; and presented her research at the International Society for Humor Studies in Paris. (Oh! She's also addressed the US Air Force, Pfizer, the Mayo Clinic, and 1,197 other organizations.)

Karyn has authored six books, she is published in peer-reviewed journals, and she is an inductee into the Speaker Hall of Fame (one of only 37 women in the world). She is a contributor to two *Chicken Soup* books, and she is the author of the *What's So Funny About...?* series *(WSFA...Diabetes? WSFA...Heart Disease? WSFA...Nursing?)* She was bestowed the Lifetime Achievement Award from the Association for Applied & Therapeutic Humor. Karyn's mission in life is to improve global health through laughter, and to heal the humor impaired.

858-603-3133   KARYNBUXMAN.COM